Boost your

child's

IMMUNE SYSTEM

Boost your child's IMMUNE SYSTEM

The natural way

Anna Niec-Oszywa

ALLEN&UNWIN

For my family

Note: The nutritional advice in this book is not intended to replace the services of a trained health professional. Your child's physical condition and diagnosis may require specific modifications or precautions. Any application of the suggestions in this book are at the reader's discretion.

First published in 2001

Allen & Unwin
83 Alexander Street
Crows Nest NSW 2065
Australia
Phone: (61 2) 8425 0100
Fax: (61 2) 9906 2218
Email: info@allenandunwin.com
Web: www.allenandunwin.com

National Library of Australia
Cataloguing-in-Publication entry:

Niec-Oszywa, Anna.
Boost your child's immune system: the natural way.

Includes index.
ISBN 1 86508 510 3.

1. Immunity—Nutritional aspects. 2. Children—Nutrition.

613.2083

Printed by Griffin Press, Adelaide

10 9 8 7 6 5 4 3 2 1

Contents

Acknowledgements

I would like to thank Xyris Software for providing me with the nutrient analysis package FoodWorks Professional Edition. FoodWorks allowed for efficient nutritional analysis of recipes and foods. Thank you also to the USDA for their nutritional data on vitamin E, selenium and copper. Finally, a special thank you to my sister Catherine for her help with data entry.

Note on recommended nutrient intakes

Approximately 40 countries have recommendations in place for the optimum daily consumption of nutrients in our diet. Official recommendations for this daily nutrient intake varies from country to country as each country has its own nutrient standards set out by the relevent expert committies.

In Australia, the recommended nutrient intakes are set by the National Health and Medical Research Council (NH&MRC) and are termed 'Recommended Dietary Intakes' or RDIs. The RDIs are the levels of essential nutrients considered adequate to meet the nutritional needs of most healthy individuals (NHMRC 1991).

In the United States the term 'Recommended Dietary Allowances' (RDAs) is the equivalent and 'Recommended Daily Amounts' are used in the United Kingdom.

While the recommendations for nutrient intakes vary between countries, the recommendations for most nutrients are similar. I have used the Australian RDIs for all calculations and references, unless otherwise stated.

Introduction

The immune system allows us to remain healthy in a world crowded with bacteria, viruses, fungi and other infectious microbes. Every day the immune system fights off foreign invaders to keep our bodies healthy. It does so through the interaction of many cells guided by numerous chemical messengers.

This system has its own recognition mechanism with cells called phagocytes, natural killer cells and mast cells keeping guard and trying to contain infections when they first take a foothold. These are helped by the T lymphocytes, which circulate in the blood and lymph around the body and keep a lookout for any foreign and unwelcome visitors. B lymphocytes are able to stage a swift attack by producing antibodies to disarm the germs and prevent them from spreading.

The T lymphocytes, (T cells, for short) work inside the cells and guard their interior. They are able to call on other cells for help as well as fight off infections by using chemical warfare. Sometimes they will destroy an entire cell that has been infected with a virus to prevent the virus from spreading. The interaction between the cells involved in the fight against germs (from now on referred to as 'fighter cells') is coordinated by cytokines. Cytokines are molecules which act as messengers between the fighter cells and which sometimes prevent the spread of infections themselves by, for example, stopping the multiplication of viruses.

Finally, it is important to mention that the immune system is classified into the innate immune system and the adaptive immune system. Innate or natural immunity is something we are born with, while an adaptive immune system evolves as we mature.

Children, particularly young children, are more susceptible to infections than adults, for two reasons. First, children are born with a natural immunity but lack an adaptive immune system. Their immune system is immature because adaptive immunity needs time to develop; it actually gains strength from previous encounters with germs. Each time an infectious germ enters the body it primes the immune system to store the information in a file and remember the encounter for the next time. This allows the immune system to stage a much more powerful attack against this particular germ should it try its luck again. So it stands to reason that very young children who have had no or very few infections have an adaptive immune system that is less mature than adults who have battled through many more infections and hardened their defences.

A second reason why children suffer more infections more often than adults, particularly upper respiratory infections, is because they come into close contact with germs. Young children discover their world by using their senses and one of the ways they do this is to place things in their mouths. Food goes in there, naturally, but so do toys, clothes, shoes, even stones and leaves, and with these come the unseen germs. Playgrounds and childcare centres make it easy for germs to pass from one child to the next. Children often catch colds and other respiratory infections from one another. Childhood is naturally a time of increased exposure to infections.

Because childhood is a time of increased vulnerability and

heightened exposure to infections it is most important to care for your children by strengthening their immune system. In the last 30 years many studies have established a link between poor nutrition and a weakened immune system, especially in children. Nutrition plays an important role in strengthening and boosting children's immune systems, which may become worn out by recurrent infections. Deficiencies in your child's supply of nutrients can manifest themselves in frequent upper respiratory tract infections, a result of weakened immunity. Whether or not children succumb to infections depends largely on the state of their immune system; this is true for both natural and adaptive immunity.

Poor nutrition leads to a poor immune response with lower levels of fighter cells, making them less efficient at fighting germs. When children eat poorly their fighter cells produce fewer antibodies, and the production of the messenger molecules that coordinate the fighter cells slows down. An inadequate diet affects every aspect of a child's immunity, from recognition of the invading germs to their coordinated destruction and finally to the gobbling up of dead germ matter by body cells called phagocytes.

Recent research has shown that during infections certain nutrients are used up at a faster rate than usual, and replenishing these is a priority to boost the immune system and prevent recurrent infections in children. The key nutrients involved in optimising children's immunity are the trace minerals zinc, iron, selenium and copper; the vitamins A, C and E; and plant-derived chemicals called flavonoids.

Protein and sufficient kilojoules are essential for the overall maintenance and running of the immune components. Children are more vulnerable to a lack of dietary protein because their needs are high during growth and development. Although a typical Western diet is high in protein, the number of children filling up on refined overprocessed carbohydrate snacks is on the rise, and these snacks leave little room for nutritious meals adequate in protein.

Similarly, eating too few kilojoules is not usually a worry in these days of plenty, although some groups of children are poor eaters while others are placed on low-fat diets too early. There are health implications for children who are placed on unsupervised low-fat diets which cut down their kilojoule intake, one of which is a depressed immunity. Eating too few kilojoules reduces the immune system's ability to act swiftly and effectively.

Low-fat diets may also predispose children to a diet low in vitamin A. Vitamin A is vital for maintaining the health of the cells that line the respiratory tract. Its deficiency in children manifests itself in more frequent respiratory infections.

Iron and zinc are two trace minerals crucial to a well functioning immune system. Children are more susceptible to iron deficiency anaemia as their growth demands a relatively greater supply of iron from their diets. It is clear that not all sources of iron are the same and that many dietary constituents affect its absorption. Zinc's absorption is also variable, depending on its food source. It is important to plan children's meals to include sufficient amounts of readily absorbed iron as well as zinc because even a mild deficiency results in compromised immunity.

Antioxidants—which include the vitamins C and E, the trace minerals selenium and copper, and plant-derived flavonoids—offer protection against free radicals. These are highly reactive molecules capable of damaging healthy fighter cells and the messenger molecules of the immune system. In the most recent Australian National Nutrition Survey (1995) children's diets were found to be low in fruit and vegetables, which are the main sources of antioxidants. Furthermore, children consume less fruit as they grow older. Reintroducing fruit into children's diets is one quick way of increasing their consumption of immunity-boosting nutrients.

Some diets make it more difficult to eat adequate amounts of immunity-boosting nutrients. A majority of scientific reports have found the vegan diet generally too restrictive to support optimal growth and development in children, being relatively low in kilojoules and protein. The lacto-ovo-vegetarian diet and the lacto-vegetarian diet can be balanced to provide all essential nutrients as well as an adequate number of kilojoules. Yet there are some guidelines to keep in mind, and balancing vegetarian meals is essential to prevent deficiencies of the immunity-boosting nutrients iron and zinc as well as protein. The strength of vegetarian diets is their rich content of antioxidants, which protect children's immunity against free radical damage.

Probiotics have made a big entry into supermarkets with the claim that they help to maintain the health of the intestinal flora. Research into their beneficial effects suggests that they are also beneficial for the immune system. They may guard against infection by preventing harmful germs from attaching themselves to the intestinal wall and, once there, gaining entry into the bloodstream. Despite these claims, not all probiotics are of equal value and it is important to distinguish the helpful ones from the unhelpful.

Supplements that claim to boost children's immunity are readily available in local pharmacies and some supermarkets. Do they work, and are they safe? A review of the more common supplements showed some interesting findings. Some preparations include a useful mix of immunity-boosting nutrients and may be worthwhile as a short-term measure for children getting over an infection. Potential problems with nutritional supplements are poorer absorption of nutrients that are not supplemented and are therefore available in much smaller amounts, possible toxic side effects and a false sense of security, which may result in a poorer diet in the long run.

Our children are becoming less active as we enjoy the luxury of advances in transport and the transformation of physical activities into mind-stimulating electronic media. We have less time to do things as families and children are showing signs of the neglected physical culture in our society. Childhood obesity which results from poor eating habits and lack of physical activity is harmful to the immune system. A moderate amount of consistent exercise is beneficial for the immune system and there is a definite need to initiate physical activities that children like and will maintain well into adulthood, even if it takes some persuasion to start with.

Nutrition during illness is very important. Although most children will lose their appetite at this time, it is important to encourage them to take nourishment in the form of light foods or nutritious drinks. You will find many useful and practical ideas on how to go about feeding children during illness in Chapter 8. During the period just after an infection it is crucial to replenish the supply of nutrients lost as a result of the illness. This is a window of opportunity to boost the immune system of children and prevent recurrent infections.

Without further ado, let's look at boosting children's resistance against infection. We will look at each immunity-boosting nutrient in turn and, more importantly, discuss how to make sure your child eats sufficient amounts of each on a daily basis. You will find many practical hints and a selection of tasty recipes that will make feeding your children an immune-boosting diet a breeze. The recipes include guidelines to the number of servings for each recipe in the different age groups, but they are just that, guidelines.

1
Kilojoules and proteins

Kilojoules have replaced calories as the unit used to measure food energy.

Kilojoules and immunity in children

A kilojoule is not a specific nutrient for boosting immunity but rather a measure of food energy that drives all types of chemical reactions important to a healthy immunity. Children who eat too few kilojoules are often tired: if we could look inside their bodies we would see many lethargic chemical reactions that need a boost of kilojoules in order to work faster. The immune system relies on its speed to be effective against infections and that speed requires kilojoules. Too many kilojoules result in childhood obesity, which is deleterious to children's immunity. Obesity brings on many metabolic changes and some of these affect the fighter cells of the immune system. Obesity can sometimes mask poor nutrition.

We look at the role of kilojoules in children's immunity more closely later, but let's first look at the whereabouts of kilojoules in children's diets.

Foods for energy in childhood

Fats and carbohydrates are the two primary sources of energy for children.

Fats are a very concentrated source of energy and the amount children need is easily met in a balanced diet. It is trickier to meet the recommendations for the amounts of complex carbohydrate. Foods rich in complex carbohydrate are relatively bulky—rice, pasta, breads and potato, for example—and the small size of a child's stomach makes it a little more difficult to consume these foods in large enough quantities. Yet these foods come packed with sustainable energy and many other nutritional goodies, so a good mix of complex carbohydrate foods is a worthwhile goal. It is a goal that is readily achieved as long as complex carbohydrates are provided at each meal throughout the day.

Children don't need high-fat diets to meet their energy needs. A slightly higher intake of fat (compared to the recommendations for adults) is acceptable, and may be needed for young children to help meet their energy needs and fuel a healthy immune system. While the recommendation for adults is that a maximum of 30% of energy should come from fats, for young children this figure may go up to 35% fat. Children, as well as adults, will benefit more from monounsaturated fats, which are found in olive and canola oils, and in margarines made from these oils. Avocados, and some nuts (almonds, cashews, hazelnuts. peanuts) are also excellent sources of monounsaturated fat and can be used as spreads on bread and toast for children.

Having looked at the whereabouts of kilojoules in children's diets, let's consider what happens when kilojoules are in short supply. It helps to remember that the immune system is a very dynamic system with fighter cells being made to order at short notice and lots of chemical energy being required for its many chemical reactions to occur. Many studies have shown the deleterious effect of insufficient kilojoules, and the poor overall nutrition in children in developing countries around the world. These reports of kilojoule and protein malnutrition paint a clear picture of compromised immunity and the many infections these children suffer as a consequence.

A deficit of kilojoules in children's diets affects the entire immune system. If significant it suppresses the normal function of the thymus gland, which is responsible for the production of T-type fighter cells and the messenger cells that coordinate the numerous cells of the immune system. The spleen, responsible for the removal of aged fighter cells and the leftover debris of infectious bugs, is also affected—in fact, it actually shrinks in size. The consequences of these and other metabolic changes are fewer fighter cells, and an overall slowed-down immune system, leaving children open to opportunistic infections. The fewer kilojoules consumed the greater the likelihood of infections. Severely malnourished children suffer fatal respiratory infections and diarrhoeal diseases, which could have been prevented. The effects can sometimes be reversed by the timely reintroduction of adequate nourishment.

In developed countries like Australia the supply of foods is plentiful and kilojoule malnutrition is rare. Two groups of children, however, deserve a mention for they are more likely to be at risk of eating insufficient kilojoules. These are children who are referred to as 'fussy-eaters', and children who are placed on low-fat diets too early.

Fussy eaters

Most children at some stage of their development will earn the name of 'fussy eater'. If your child refuses to eat when you have food ready, or only nibbles at it, or seems able to last without food for ages—don't worry. Depending on the child's age and developmental stage, they may simply be establishing their independence, going through a natural food fad or responding to a slowing down in their growth rate with a diminished appetite. Cultivate patience, calmness and a quiet determination in youself as you work through these times. *Remember, there is no real problem unless your child is losing weight or is not making sufficient progress with weight or height.*

If you suspect your child is not eating enough, keeping an eye on their weight is a good idea. To record weight accurately, weigh your child first thing in the morning using the same scales on the same surface.

It may be difficult to notice weight loss in your child if it happens very gradually. If you suspect weight loss, weigh your child over a period of time, twice weekly, and look at the trend in the weight. Don't make an issue of weight but explain to children who are old enough to understand that you are weighing them to make sure they are growing up healthy and strong. Have a brief talk about food and how certain foods make them strong and tall. If your child likes sport tell them they will have more energy to play the sport they like for longer. This brief talk will often enthuse a youngster to eat more, even if only for a little while.

Other hints to persuade your child to eat:

- Keep offering new foods time and time again, as research shows that it takes eight to ten offerings before a new food is accepted. Most parents tend to give up after two or three tries.
- Mix new foods with old favourites.
- Encourage new tastes, but don't force.
- Don't fall into the habit of thinking the next meal or snack is not far-away and take food away without trying your best to tempt your child.
- Don't fall into the trap of offering sweets as a last resort.

- Involve your child with food preparation and make it fun.
- Above all, relax—try talking about pleasant things and not food worries.
- Switching off the TV at mealtimes helps, as it can be a distraction.

It helps to know that one study found a similar number of parents and children who admitted to being fussy eaters, about 22% for both!

Finally, be on the lookout for medical conditions that could be causing poor appetite, for example, malabsorption of lactose (a sugar in milk). Visit your doctor or find a dietitian for further help if you are concerned that this may be the case. Read through the following section for useful hints on how to increase the kilojoules in your child's diet without asking the child to eat *more* food.

Making each bite count a little more

In times of fussy eating children will benefit from extra kilojoules per mouthful. You can add extra kilojoules to the meals just before serving in such a way that they don't increase the overall bulk of the meal. Remember that boosting kilojoules for poor eaters is boosting their immune system. Here is how.

- *Monounsaturated spreads, oil and mayonnaise.* Add to pureed foods, vegetables, sandwiches, casseroles, soups, rice and pasta. These additions go with almost everything and provide 150–170 kilojoules per teaspoon.
- *Powdered milk.* Excellent with smoothies, milkshakes, mashed potato, cooked cereals and yoghurt. One tablespoon provides 100 kilojoules.
- *Grated cheese.* Grated mozzarella cheese or grated mature cheese, like cheddar, is good for topping rice, pasta, fish, vegetables,

scrambled eggs, casseroles and soups. Each 30 grams provides 420 kilojoules.

- *Peanut butter.* Makes a great spread on some vegetables for older children. May be used freely on toast pieces, crackers, muffins for children of all ages—just vary bite size and thickness. For toddlers use smooth peanut butter. Provides 420 kilojoules per tablespoon.
- *Avocado.* Spread on toast, bread, crackers; add to sandwiches. Each quarter of avocado gives about 315 kilojoules.
- *Nuts.* Ground nuts can be added to ice-cream, yoghurt, custard and baked goods, and sprinkled on cereal for children of all ages. Whole nuts can be given to children from the age of five. One tablespoon of ground almonds (almond meal) has about 230 kilojoules.
- *Wheat germ.* Wheat germ can be added to homemade goodies such as pancakes, biscuits, muffins and breads; also goes well with cooked cereal. One tablespoon of wheat germ contains about 100 kilojoules.

Note that these guidelines are general. Avoid feeding peanuts or dairy products to children allergic to these foods.

The implications of low-fat diets in early childhood

The second group of children more susceptible to getting insufficient kilojoules are those children less than five years of age who are placed on very low-fat diets that exclude eggs, severely limit lean meats and include skim milk, with or without other low-fat products. Such low-fat diets are not suitable for children under five years of age. They have been shown to be low in kilojoules, as well as in vitamin E, a fat-soluble vitamin that is very important for a healthy immune system (we look at vitamin E later).

Some small but significant studies have shown that undue fat restriction results in low body weight and height, and leads to stunting in children. The stunting is reversible if caught during the growing stage by relaxing the fat restriction and thus increasing the kilojoules.

There is insufficient scientific evidence to support very low-fat diets in childhood as a preventive measure against heart disease in later stages of life. The available evidence is incomplete and shows no clear connection between a moderate fat intake in childhood and increased rates of atherosclerosis in adulthood.

If you are concerned about heart disease because of a strong family history, remember that monounsaturated fats don't increase the risk of heart disease; they do provide a young child with the much needed kilojoules for a robust immune system. So rather than restricting fat in your child's diet, use more monounsaturated fat and less saturated fat. Sources of monounsaturated fats include olive oil, canola oil, avocado, hazelnuts, cashews and peanuts (remember to grind these for young children).

Saturated fats include all animal fats plus coconut fat and some processed vegetable fat.

Excess body weight in children

Excess body weight slows children down, and their immune system as well. Children who consume too many kilojoules—mostly from eating too much fat and/or sugar—gain weight too rapidly and the excess kilojoules consumed have a negative effect on their immune system.

In developed countries like Australia, overweight rather than underweight has become the health risk for children. This is a reflection of a food supply with a high percentage of processed foods that are high in fat or sugar, or both. Children's diets today are more likely to contain higher amounts of sugar, saturated fat and refined foods with low nutritional value. These excess kilojoules result in excess weight which has been shown to have a negative effect on children's immunity.

Numerous studies show that obesity lowers the body's resistance to infections. Studies with children show that obese children are more prone to respiratory infections than children whose weight is within the healthy weight percentile. The reasons for this effect are not known, although one study pointed at poor nutrition as the answer. This study looked at the immunity of obese children attending a weight-loss clinic and showed that, in comparison with children with normal weight, obese children had a less robust immune system. Their immune systems were less able to fight off bacteria, as well as being slower off the mark.

The reseachers then looked at the children's iron and zinc levels in the two groups and compared the results for these two nutrients. They found that the children with a slower and less efficient immune system were more likely to have low iron and/or zinc levels, and that these children came mostly from the obese group. The study concluded that the immunity of children is reduced as a consequence of poor nutrition, particularly poor intakes of the micronutrients zinc and iron.

It would be premature to jump to the conclusion that all overweight children are poorly nourished and are therefore more likely to suffer from respiratory and other infections. I can, however, see this happening in a subgroup of children whose eating habits are poor in general as a result of eating high-energy foods with little other nutritional value. Nutritionists call this eating 'empty' kilojoules. The consequence of such eating habits in children, as in adults, is weight gain coupled with hidden inadequate nutrition. This type of obesity goes hand in hand with compromised immunity. It is very important to recognise that 'big'—as in overweight—does not mean healthy.

It is equally important, however, that children are not placed on diets. Undue kilojoule restriction in children does more harm than good. Children's weight loss, if needed, should be supervised by a health professional trained in children's nutritional needs and the program should proceed at a slow and gradual rate so as not to impair growth. A study of obese children who dieted for four weeks found that *fast weight-loss diets,* even for a short time, result in a significant decrease in the number of fighter cells.

To reduce your child's weight gradually or simply to allow children to 'grow into' their weight, reduce saturated fats in your child's diet. In particular, look out for foods that are high in saturated fat but have little nutritional value. These are all types of highly processed crisps, chips, fatty crackers and biscuits. Target these first, and replace with more nutritious snacks like raisin toast, low-fat fruit muffins, yoghurts and fruit smoothies. In your cooking, remove excess meat fat and poultry skin. Take care with cold cuts like salami, devon and any processed high-fat meats and substitute lean plain meats, dressing them with mustards, small amounts of mint jelly or cranberry sauce. Include reduced-fat dairy products in your child's diet if there is obesity. Don't forget to look at drinks and to limit or avoid soft drinks that are high in sugar and a source of empty kilojoules. When making changes don't single out the child but involve the entire family as much as possible.

Children's energy needs

Having looked at the two extremes of kilojoule intake and their deleterious consequences on the immune system, we'll now look at how much energy is optimal for children. The answer is easy—it is the number of kilojoules that sustains their growth and development at the right pace.

To find out if your child is growing well and putting on a healthy amount of weight, use the growth and development charts at the end of this chapter. The most practical way is to plot your child's growth on the chart and compare it with the percentile lines for both weight and height according to the age and gender of your child. It is best to plot weight and height on the charts concurrently to see the progress of your child's development.

If your child's growth is healthy, you will see that if you draw a line between the points you have plotted, the line will run along, or parallel to, one of the percentile bands. If you see an irregular pattern or a sudden levelling off then providing there was no mistake in your measurements or plotting, your child is not growing to his or her full potential. If that is the case, consult your doctor or a dietitian to reassess your child's diet and development.

Growth and development charts need to be completed over a period of time to give you a proper indication of whether or not your child is eating sufficient food. You can use the charts at the end of the chapter as a starting point. If you need an answer more quickly, take a look at the recommended number of serves from the five different food groups and the quantities making up each serve.

The five food groups are:

- breads and cereals
- fruit and vegetables
- meats and alternatives
- milk and dairy
- fats including oils, margarine and butter.

Energy needs on a daily basis

Relative to their body size the kilojoule needs of children are greater than those of adults. Energy requirements relative to the child's size are highest in the first five years of life. They peak in the toddler years, and generally decrease with age. For all children, and especially young children, it can be quite difficult to obtain sufficient energy as their stomachs are relatively small at a time of rapid growth and development. This is one of the reasons why children need their own dietary guidelines. Table 1.1 sets out the recommended daily amounts from the five food groups.

Proteins for robust immunity

Proteins are essential for a robust immune system. They are often called the 'building blocks of life'. Proteins make up a myriad of body parts small and large, from elastic skin fibres to firm-textured hair and nails. They are involved in many crucial reactions as enzymes or chemical messengers, and form many transport molecules in our blood. The usefulness of proteins comes from their special structure. Each protein is made up of a unique sequence of amino acids that can be likened to a sequence of different-coloured beads on a necklace. There are 23 amino acids which can be put together in countless ways to produce different types of proteins.

Proteins, or protein structures, are involved in many ways in the immune system. The immune system is made up of numerous fighter cells and their artillery which, in turn, are made mostly out of proteins. These components are used and destroyed on a regular basis so there is a constant need to rejuvenate the protein-rich components. Depending on your children's eating habits, they may or may not consume enough protein-rich foods to support a healthy immune system. Nine amino acids, called essential amino acids, are particularly important for children as they cannot be made by any other means.

Children's protein needs are greater than those of adults because extra protein is needed for healthy growth and development.

Table 1.1

Recommended daily serves from the five food groups, by age

1. Breads and Cereals	Four to six servings daily		
	1–3 years	*4–7 years*	*8–11 years*
Bread	1/2–1 slice	1 slice	1–2 slices
Cooked cereals, rice and pasta	1/4–1/3 cup	1/2 cup	1/2–3/4 cup
Ready to eat cereal	1/2 cup	1/2 cup	3/4–1 cup
2. Vegetables and Fruit	Three to five servings of vegetables; two to four servings of fruit daily		
	1–3 years	*4–7 years*	*8–11 years*
Vitamin C sources Citrus fruit, berries, peppers, tomatoes, broccoli, cauliflower, cabbage	1/4 cup	1/4 cup	1/2 cup
Vitamin A sources Apricots, peaches, melons, carrots, spinach, squash, pumpkin	1/4 cup	1/4 cup	1/2 cup
Other	1/4 cup	1/4 cup	1/2 cup
3. Milk and Dairy	Three to four servings daily		
	1–3 years	*4–7 years*	*8–11 years*
Milk	150 ml	150 ml	1 cup
Soy milk, fortified	150 ml	150 ml	1 cup
Yoghurt	100 g	150 g	200 g
Cheese	30 g	30 g	30 g
Custard	1/2 cup	1/2 cup	1 cup
4. Meat and Alternatives	Two or more servings		
	1–3 years	*4–7 years*	*8–11 years*
Meat/poultry, lean	35 g	45 g	65 g
Fish	40 g	50 g	75 g
Eggs	1	1	2
Peanut butter	1 tblsp	1 tblsp	2 tblsp
Baked beans	1/4 cup	1/2 cup	1 cup
5. Fats	Two serves or as needed to boost kilojoules		
	1–3 years	*4–7 years*	*8–11 years*
Monounsaturated fats	1 teaspoon	1 teaspoon	2 teaspoons

Children need more protein per kilogram of body weight than adults. Children are more vulnerable to a lack of dietary protein because of their needs so it is important to provide them with sufficient dietary protein on a daily basis. A shortage of good quality protein in children's diets rapidly reduces the performance of the immune system. Children's defences against bacteria in particular will crumble as there will be insufficient amino acids to make antibodies against the invading microbes.

It is worrying to hear reports of children's diets being high in fat and sugar because filling up on sweet, fatty foods leaves little room for good quality, nutritious protein choices. Adults can eat a high-fat, high-sugar diet and still eat enough protein while young children have a smaller appetite because of their smaller stomach volume and it is more difficult to meet their protein needs if they indulge too often in sweets, crisps and other high-energy, low protein foods.

Sources and quality of proteins

Where do we turn for protein in the diet and what are the best food sources? Are all protein sources of equal value?

The best sources of proteins are fish, chicken, lean meats, eggs and dairy foods. They have the highest content of protein per weight and the quality of protein is superior to the proteins found in plant foods. The proteins in fish, chicken, meats, eggs and dairy products are of high biological value and are referred to as *complete* proteins. They are 'complete' because they contain the entire set of amino acids and they will provide your child with all the raw materials needed to make any body protein.

The proteins found in foods of plant origin, with the exception of soybeans, lack balance in the amino acids they provide and are called 'incomplete' for that reason. Depending on the source, plant proteins lack one or several amino acids from the complete set. Fortunately, with some clever food combining this shortcoming of plant proteins may be overcome. It is, however, important to plan your child's diet carefully if you do decide to care for the child's nutritional needs with a diet based mostly on plant foods.

- The diet of *omnivores* includes fish, chicken, meat, eggs and dairy products—all excellent sources of good quality proteins. With this diet it is usually not difficult to provide your child with adequate protein.
- A vegetarian diet including eggs and milk—called a *lacto-ovo vegetarian* diet—can be made nutritionally balanced for your child with some forward planning.
- In a strict vegetarian diet that excludes all foods of animal origin —a *vegan* diet—legumes, nuts and soybean products like tofu are the best sources of proteins. I do not recommend a strict vegan diet for young children as they find it very difficult to eat sufficient amounts of plant foods to meet their protein and kilojoule needs. Children's stomachs are small and little can be eaten at any one time. It is important to provide children with food rich in nutrients and good quality proteins to optimise growth and development and support a robust immunity.

If you are looking after your child's nutrition with a vegetarian diet, Chapter 7 offers many useful hints to help you balance a vegetarian diet so as to provide your child with adequate nutrition for a healthy immune system.

Children's protein needs—how much is optimum?

The protein needs of children vary depending on their age.

Toddlers aged 1–3 years need 14–18 grams of protein daily. Another way of working out the daily protein needs of children in this age group is to multiply the child's weight in kilograms by 1.5. This will give the number of protein grams to provide daily. For example, if a child weighs 12 kilograms, $12 \times 1.5 = 18$. So a 12-kilogram toddler needs around 18 grams of protein daily.

Young children aged 4–7 years need 18–24 grams of protein daily. Or you can work out the daily protein needs of children in this age group by multiplying the child's weight by 1.4. This will give the number of protein grams needed daily. For example, for a child weighing 15 kilograms, $15 \times 1.4 = 21$. So for a 15-kilogram child in this age group the protein needs are around 21 grams daily.

Older children 8–11 years: in this age group the protein needs for girls and boys are almost identical. For both, the recommended amount of protein to be eaten daily is in the range 27–39 grams.

How do the recommended amounts of protein translate into food choices? What are the best food choices in each age group and what is a good combination for children? The following sections will guide you through the answers. Let's start with the protein content of some useful protein-rich foods.

Protein content of foods

In the five food groups the protein content of foods varies tremendously.

The highest amounts of protein are found in the Meat and Alternatives food group, and in the Milk and Dairy food group. In Tables 1.2 and 1.3 you will find the amounts of protein in grams for numerous foods in these two food groups. The serves are smaller than those recommended for adults because children have smaller stomachs and their total protein needs are less.

Meeting children's daily protein needs

We now look in detail at meal planning to meet the daily protein needs of three different age groups: toddlers, children 4–7 years and older children aged 8–11 years.

Table 1.2

Protein content of foods in the Meat and Alternatives group

Food	Quantity	Protein (grams)
Meats	30 g	7
Poultry	30 g	7
Fish	30 g	7
Eggs	60 g	8
Cooked legumes	1/2 cup	6
Tofu	40 g	5
Peanut butter	1 tblsp	7
Nuts*	30 g	6

* Don't offer whole or cracked nuts to children under the age of five as they may choke. Instead, add ground nuts and almond meal to their foods (see recipes for some great ideas).
Source: FoodWorks Professional Edition, Copyright 1998–2000 Xyris Software.

Table 1.3

Protein content of foods in the Milk and Dairy group

Food	Quantity	Protein (grams)
Milk	150 ml	5
Yoghurt	100 ml	5
Cheese, mature*	30 g	8
Ricotta	1/4 cup	7
Cottage cheese, creamed	1/4 cup	9
Custard	150 ml	6
Ice-cream	1/2 cup	3

* Cheddar, Swiss, edam etc.
Source: FoodWorks Professional Edition, Copyright 1998–2000 Xyris Software.

Toddlers

Eating time between 12 and 36 months of age is a fast learning curve for young children. They begin by being clumsy and messy while trying to eat with their fingers, then achieve more co-ordinated movements and are able to eat with a bowl and spoon, and finally reach the stage of being able to eat off a plate with a fork. During this time they discover different food textures but they are still too young to eat hard or brittle foods and prefer simple foods to mixtures. It is also a time when children begin to exert their independence and display food likes and dislikes.

Food fads are a natural part of feeding a toddler. Although food fads are natural, if not supervised the diets of toddlers may become overly limited with little food variety, placing the child at risk of nutrient deficiencies. Offer a wide variety of protein-rich foods and allow the child to select from within these choices.

Because toddlers and young children have small tummies relative to their size they need more frequent meals than adults. I recommend three main meals with two or three between-meal snacks. Make the between-meal snacks nourishing and interesting. Add interest by using different tastes, colours and shapes of foods.

The texture of meat

Unlike dairy products and eggs, the other sources of protein in the diet have a tough texture in the mouth of the toddler. Some children refuse meats or chicken because they quickly tire of chewing.

Eating meat is a habit that young children have to learn, and lessons should start fairly early. At about eight months children are introduced to pureed meats and this acts as a gradual introduction to more textured meats. They can move to soft lumps as in minced meat to more solid cubes in casseroles and finally to soft roast and grilled meats.

If your child refuses red meat and chicken, try preparing the meat in different ways so as to vary the texture and see whether this makes a difference. Once you find a texture the child is happy with you can gradually return to the foods that offer the most appropriate texture for the child's age. Be patient, and innovate with colour to add interest to meals. You may find the delicious and colourful recipes at the end of this chapter helpful.

Daily protein needs of a toddler

Here is a daily protein plan for children aged 1–3 years.

Children in this age group need 14–18 grams of protein daily, but remember that these are *minimum* daily amounts. If we divide up this amount it works out to 3–4 grams of protein at the three main meals and 2–4 gram protein snacks between the meals, depending on whether your child has two or three snacks during the day. By ensuring that your children have protein at each meal and for most snacks they are unlikely to miss out on their daily protein needs.

Remember, however, that children's appetites vary greatly from meal to meal and day to day, and they may eat better at one meal than the next. If you notice your child's appetite is poor at one meal, try to make up the protein that has been missed later in the day by providing a larger than usual protein-rich snack. You will find that your child's overall protein intake will be adequate as long as you continue to offer protein-rich foods—don't offer carbohydrate-rich foods such as instant noodles or rice, only because children will readily fill up on these without getting adequate protein for their needs.

It's even more damaging to the protein intake of young children if they are allowed to snack on fatty and sugary foods such as chocolate or cake. This habit will predispose children to fill up on kilojoule-dense foods that have little protein. Sweets, in particular, dull children's appetites—if eaten before main meals they will almost certainly result in refusal to eat the protein-rich foods served at these meals.

To provide the right amount of protein for your toddler to ensure healthy growth and development and a healthy immune system, start with the basic food amounts given below. First, the protein portions for main meals—each provides a minimum of 4 grams of protein.

Breakfast examples

- ½ cup regular cow's milk
- ½ cup calcium-fortified soy milk
- 45 g egg
- ¼ cup baked beans
- 3 teaspoons smooth peanut butter

Lunch examples

- 2 tablespoons fresh ricotta cheese
- 2 tablespoons fresh cottage cheese
- 20 g or thin slice of ham, turkey, shaved chicken
- 15 g tasty cheese or other mature cheese
- 50 g tofu

Dinner examples

- 20 g fish
- 20 g cooked meats
- 20 g cooked chicken or turkey
- 2 tablespoons bolognaise sauce
- ¼ cup cooked legumes

Between-meal snacks to provide your toddler with a minimum of 4 grams of protein:

- ½ cup regular cow's milk
- ½ cup soy beverage
- 100 ml smooth yoghurt
- 200 ml fruit smoothie
- ½ cup custard

Between-meal snacks to provide your toddler with a minimum of 2 grams of protein:

- fresh fruit pieces and 3 tablespoons smooth yoghurt
- ¼ cup fromage frais

- ½ small banana and ¼ cup custard
- 1 pikelet with ½ small banana
- ⅓ cup ice-cream
- ½ slice wholemeal bread with 1 teaspoon smooth peanut butter
- ½ slice wholemeal bread with 1 tablespoon cottage or ricotta cheese

Hints to help your toddler eat protein-rich foods

- Arrange regular mealtimes so your child is not too tired to eat.
- Offer small portions first and offer second helpings if liked.
- Serve between-meal snacks at least an hour before a main meal.
- Keep sweets out of sight until savoury foods are eaten.
- Don't offer sweet drinks or fruit juice just before a main meal.

Children aged 4–7 years

From four years onwards chilren aquire the skills of self-feeding and shift more of their attention to food. They become more interested in food, will often ask questions about it and will begin to request their favourite foods. Plain foods are still preferred to mixtures, although children at this age are more willing to try new foods. It is also a time when peer pressure becomes important, and television and friends will influence children's choices. Once children reach school age the influence of their peers becomes even more important as they compare lunches and visit the school canteen. It is important to provide school lunches and snacks that are rich in protein.

Daily protein plan for children aged 4–7 years

Children in this age group need 18–24 grams of protein daily. Remember, these are *minimum* daily amounts. If we divide up this amount it works out at 4–6 grams of protein at each main meal and 2–4 gram protein snacks between the meals, depending on whether your child has two or three snacks during the day. By ensuring that your children have protein at each meal and for most snacks they are unlikely to miss out on their daily protein needs.

Remember that children's appetites may still vary somewhat from one day to the next although this is less likely after the toddler years are over. If you notice your child's appetite is poor at one meal, try to make up the protein that has been missed later in the day—you could provide an extra protein-rich snack, or offer a larger than usual snack. You will find that, overall, your child's protein intake will be adequate as long as you continue to offer protein-rich foods—don't offer carbohydrate-rich foods such as instant noodles or rice, only because children will readily fill up on these without getting adequate protein for their needs. Limit sweets and never offer them before a main meal as they will spoil your child's appetite.

To provide the right amount of protein for children in this age group to ensure healthy growth and development and a healthy immune system, start with these basic food amounts. Each portion example provides a minimum of 6 grams of protein.

Breakfast

- 3/4 cup regular cow's milk
- 3/4 cup calcium-fortified soy milk
- 60 g egg
- 1/2 cup baked beans
- I tablespoon smooth peanut butter

Lunch

- 1/4 cup fresh ricotta cheese
- 1/4 cup cottage cheese
- 30 g ham, turkey or shaved chicken
- standard slice of tasty cheese or other mature cheese
- small baked potato and 20 g tasty cheese
- 80 g tofu

Dinner

- 40 g fish
- 35 g cooked meats
- 35 g cooked chicken
- 2 tablespoons bolognaise sauce
- ½ cup cooked legumes (e.g. lentils, dried beans)

Between-meal snacks to provide a minimum of 4 grams of protein:

- 100 ml regular cow's milk
- 100 ml fortified soy beverage
- 100 ml yoghurt
- ¼ cup fromage frais
- 1 cup fruit smoothie

Between-meal snacks to provide a minimum of 2 grams of protein:

- fresh fruit pieces and 3 tablespoons yoghurt
- ½ small banana and ¼ cup custard
- 1 pikelet with ½ small banana
- ⅓ cup ice-cream
- ½ slice wholemeal bread with 1 teaspoon peanut butter
- ½ slice bread with 1 tablespoon cottage or ricotta cheese

Daily protein plan for children aged 8–11 years

In this age group the protein needs for girls and boys are almost identical. For both, the recommended daily amount of protein is 27–39 grams. Meeting the protein needs of older children is much easier for they are now able to eat larger amounts at one meal and can, therefore, catch up more quickly if they fail to eat sufficient protein at any one meal. Follow these guidelines to provide your child with enough protein in the daily diet.

Offer a nutritious breakfast, aiming for approximately 10 grams of protein. This can be made up from one of the following:

- 2 small eggs on toast
- 30 g cereal with 200 ml milk
- one slice of toast with cheese and one slice of toast with vegemite

Children in this age group are at risk of developing the habit of skipping breakfast and opting for a snack or a fast meal on the way to school with their peers. Some will skip breakfast-time eating altogether. Be attentive to any signs of this happening in your child and reinforce the importance of having breakfast.

Children who skip breakfast may miss out on about 30% of their daily protein needs. Depending on their food choices at school, they may or may not make up this deficit during the day.

Ensure that your child has dinner with the family and eats fish, chicken, lean meats or alternative foods rich in protein.

It is also in this age group that signs of vegetarianism or pseudo-vegetarian food preferences may first appear—only to be strengthened in adolescence. Your growing child may suddenly become reluctant to eat red meat or fish or chicken. You may hear remarks of this nature: 'This meat tastes funny' or 'I don't like chicken'. Or you may just notice a general reluctance to eat meat. Children who undertake these diet changes usually fill up on carbohydrate-rich foods like bread and noodles or processed foods such as corn chips, potato crisps and biscuits. While breads and pasta are important to a healthy diet, they are also low in protein. Children who go off meats can become deficient in protein, and their immune system may soon start to show signs of wear. They often feel tired and succumb to more infections.

Try to discuss this avoidance to work out whether it is a passing food fad or whether there is more at stake—for example, an attempt at weight loss (which may occur as early as eight years of age). Girls are more likely to cut out meat from their diet than boys in an attempt to lose weight. You may want to seek the help of an accredited dietitian if you are concerned. In all cases, continue to offer meat, chicken and fish cooked in different ways and encourage your child to eat them. If this does not help, ensure they have other foods rich in protein as substitutes in their diet.

Choose from the following:

- 65-g portion meat or poultry
- 75 g fish
- 1¼ cup cooked legumes
- two eggs
- 200 g tofu
- 1 cup nuts
- 60 g mature cheese
- ½ cup ricotta/cottage cheese

Growth and development charts

Birth–36 months: girls

Length-for-age and weight-for-age percentiles

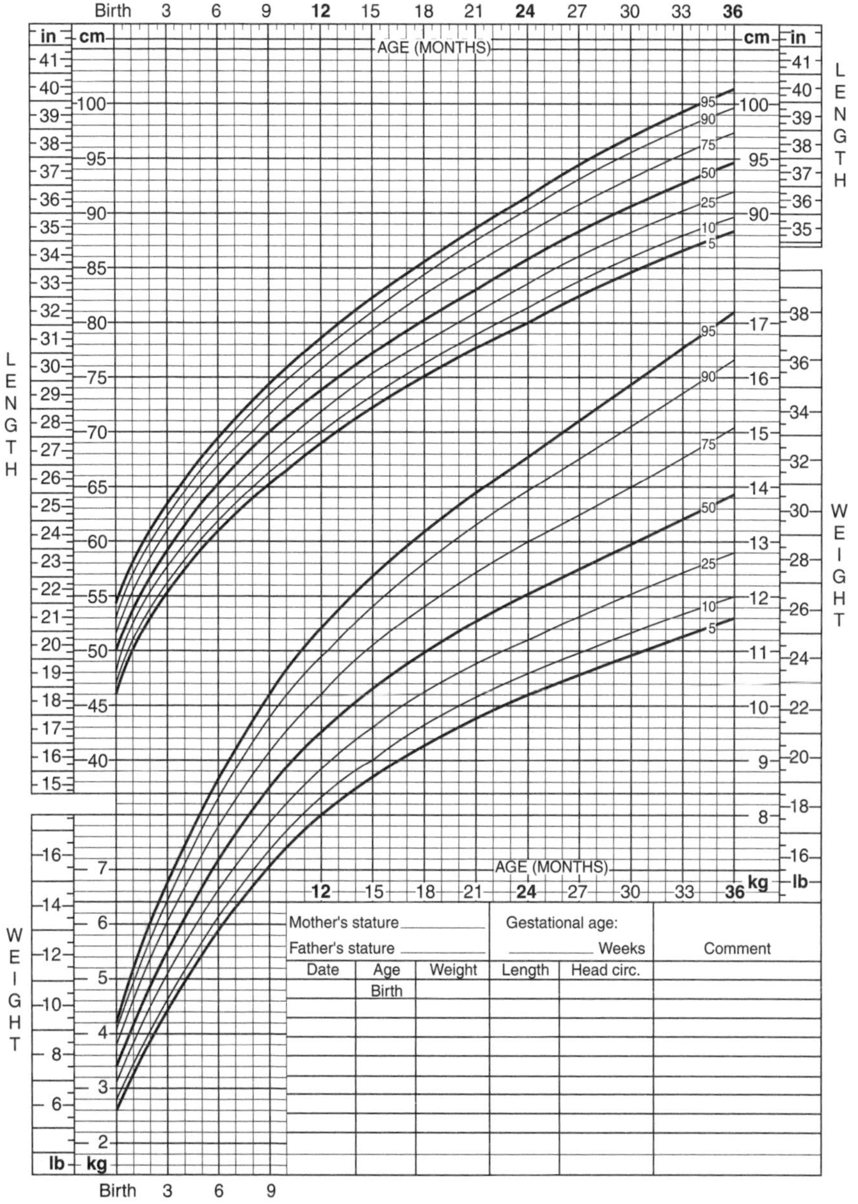

Revised 21 November 2000.

Source: Developed by the National Center for Health Statistics in collaboration with the National Center for Chronic Disease Prevention and Health Promotion (2000). **http://www.cdc.gov/growthcharts**

Growth and development charts

Birth–36 months: boys

Length-for-age and weight-for-age percentiles

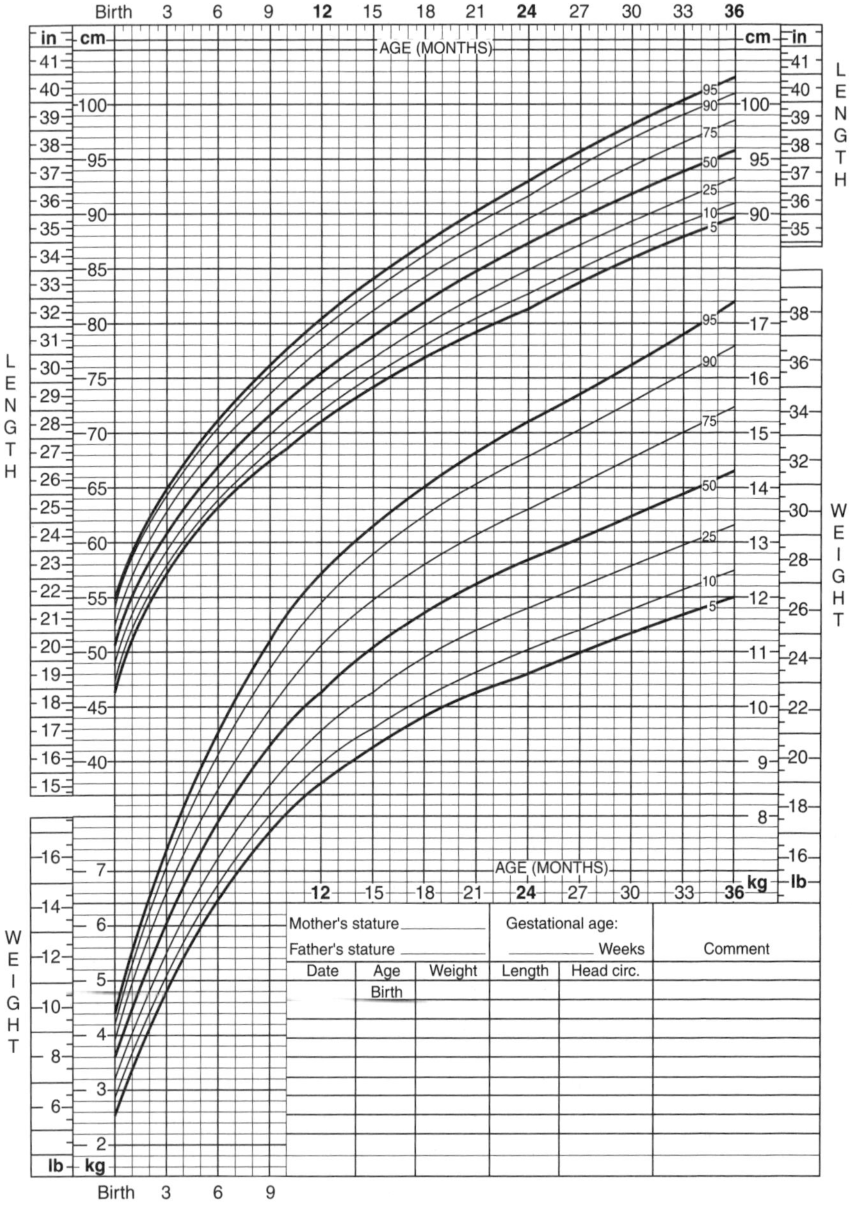

Revised 21 November 2000.

Source: Developed by the National Center for Health Statistics in collaboration with the National Center for Chronic Disease Prevention and Health Promotion (2000). **http://www.cdc.gov/growthcharts**

Growth and development charts

2–20 years: girls

Stature-for-age and weight-for-age percentiles

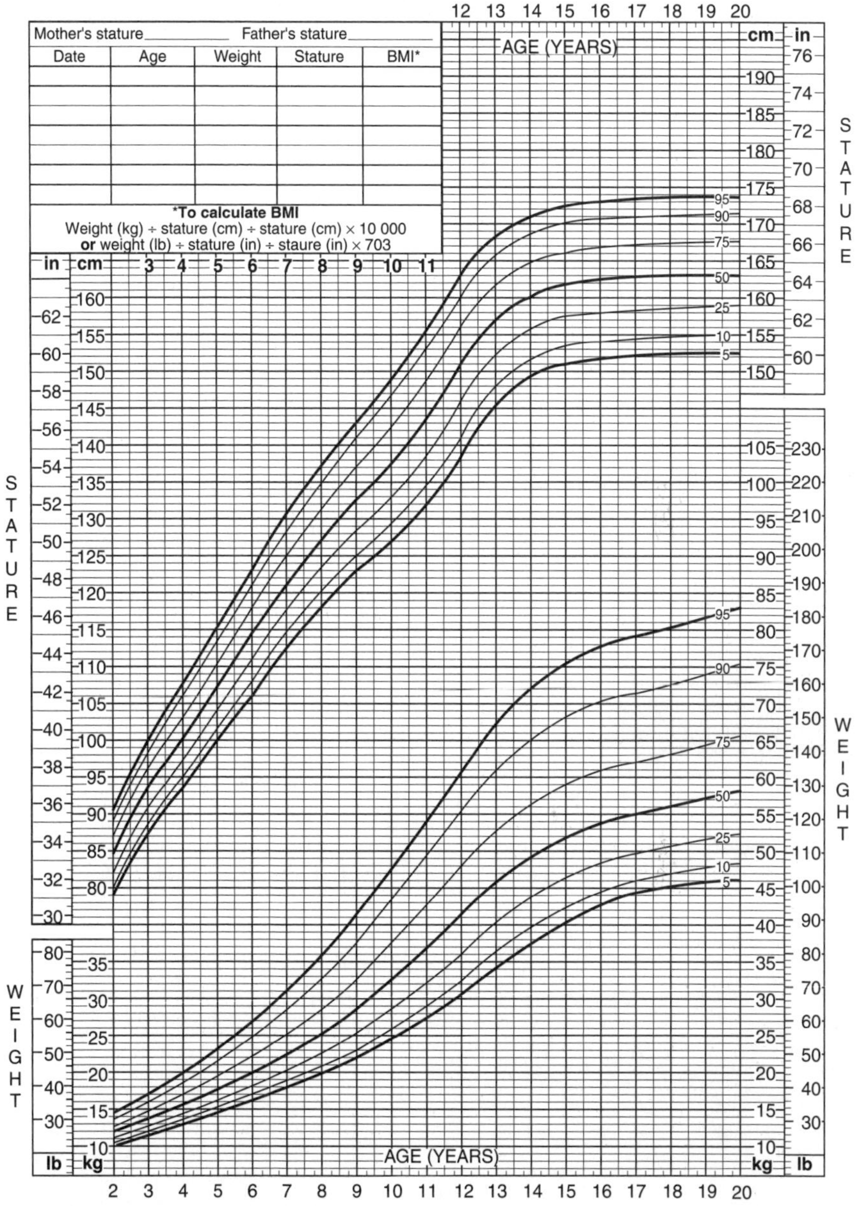

Revised and corrected 28 November 2000.

Source: Developed by the National Center for Health Statistics in collaboration with the National Center for Chronic Disease Prevention and Health Promotion (2000). **http://www.cdc.gov/growthcharts**

Growth and development charts

2–20 years: boys

Stature-for-age and weight-for-age percentiles

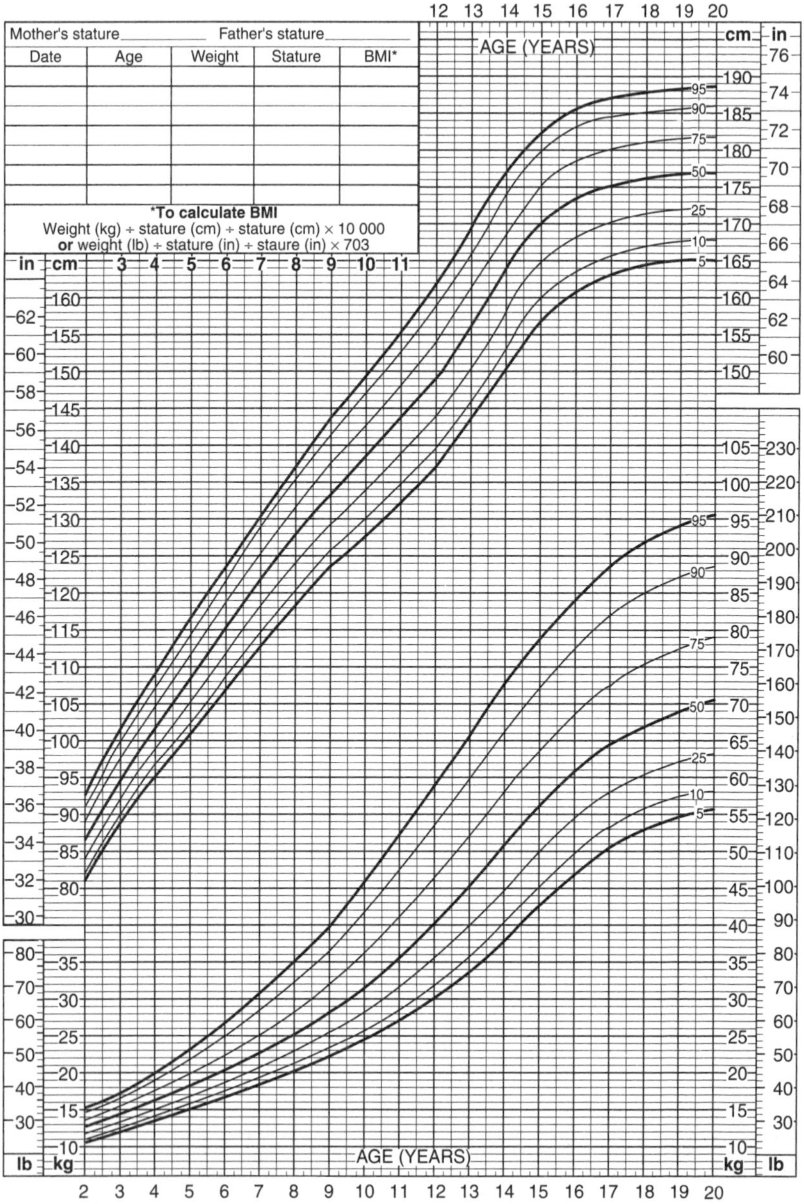

Revised and corrected 21 November 2000.

Source: Developed by the National Center for Health Statistics in collaboration with the National Center for Chronic Disease Prevention and Health Promotion (2000). **http://www.cdc.gov/growthcharts**

Ingredients

Makes approximately:
10 serves for 1–3 year olds
8 serves for 4–7 year olds
6 serves for 8–11 year olds

2 cups rice
3 cups cold water
5 tablespoons olive oil
4 large eggs, lightly beaten
1/2 cup diced onion
1 cup diced bacon (trimmed)
1/2 cup small cooked prawns
1/2 cup cooked fresh or thawed frozen peas
1/2 cup fresh or thawed corn kernels
4 spring onions, finely chopped
1 cup seeded, diced tomato
salt to taste (omit for toddlers and young children)
freshly ground black pepper to taste
1/2 cup chopped fresh basil (optional)

Method

- Rinse rice two or three times or until water runs clear, drain well.
- In a medium saucepan bring the 3 cups of water to a boil, add rice and stir once.
- Reduce heat to low and cook for 5 minutes; cover and simmer for 15 minutes or until rice is tender.
- In a large skillet, heat 4 tablespoons oil over medium-high heat.
- Add eggs and cook until lightly set, stirring with a wooden spoon to break into tiny pieces.
- Continue to cook, stirring, until eggs are lightly browned, 4 to 5 minutes.
- Remove to a small bowl with a slotted spoon and set aside.
- In the same skillet, heat the remaining tablespoon of oil, add onion and stir-fry over high heat until soft and lightly golden, about 2 minutes.
- Add bacon and prawns, peas, corn and spring onions and stir-fry until heated through, about 3 minutes.
- Add tomato and sprinkle in salt, stir in cooked rice and egg, breaking up any lumps.
- Mix well and heat through, season to taste with pepper and stir in basil.
- Serve right away.

Nutritional analysis per serve
Age 1–3 years: energy 1250 kJ—20% RDI; protein 10.0 g—55% RDI
Age 4–7 years: energy 1560 kJ—20% RDI; protein 12.5 g—50% RDI
Age 8–11 years: energy 2080 kJ—25% RDI; protein 17.0 g—45% RDI

Ingredients

Makes 1 serve

1 egg, lightly beaten

4 tablespoons milk

2 tablespoons creamed sweet corn

Method

- Cook egg mixture in non-stick frypan until just set.
- Add sweet corn and spread over one half of omelette.
- Fold one half of omelette over the other.
- Cook a further minute to warm corn through.
- Cool and serve.

Nutritional analysis per serve	Age 1–3 years: energy 720 kJ—12% RDI; protein 11 g—60% RDI Age 4–7 years: energy 720 kJ— 9% RDI; protein 11 g—47% RDI Age 8–11 years: energy 720 kJ— 9% RDI; protein 11 g—30% RDI

Grind the nuts for children under 5 years of age.

Ingredients

Makes approximately:
8 serves for 1–3 year olds
6 serves for older children

filo pastry

margarine or butter

350 g eating apples

juice of 1 lemon

50 g currants or sultanas

1 tablespoon wheat germ

25 g chopped or flaked almonds

2 teaspoons honey

2 teaspoons ground cinnamon

2 teaspoons soft margarine or butter

Method

- Heat oven to 220°C, and grease a baking sheet.
- Brush each filo sheet with margarine or butter and arrange the sheets one on top of the other.
- Slice the unpeeled apples very thinly and cut into small pieces into a bowl.
- Pour over the lemon juice and stir in the currants or sultanas, wheat germ, almonds, honey and 1 teaspoon cinnamon.
- Spread the apple mixture evenly over the pastry.
- Brush with half the melted margarine or butter.
- Roll up the pastry and transfer it to a baking sheet.
- Brush it with the remaining melted margarine or butter and sprinkle with the remaining cinnamon.
- Bake for 10 minutes, then reduce the heat to 190°C and bake for a further 20 minutes.

Nutritional analysis per serve
Age 1–3 years: energy 595 kJ—10% RDI; protein 3.5 g—20% RDI
Age 4–7 years: energy 820 kJ—10% RDI; protein 4.4 g—25% RDI
Age 8–11 years: energy 820 kJ—10% RDI; protein 4.4 g—12% RDI

Ingredients

Makes 2 serves

1 cup milk

1 tablespoon white round-grain rice

honey

cinnamon sugar

Method

- Place milk and rice in a medium saucepan.
- Cook over a medium heat for 2 minutes, cover.
- Stir once.
- Reduce heat to low and cook, covered, for 15 minutes, stirring every 2 minutes.
- Sweeten with a little honey.
- Stand for 5 minutes.
- Sprinkle with a little cinnamon sugar.

Nutritional analysis per serve	Age 1–3 years: energy 685 kJ—11% RDI; protein 5.4 g—30% RDI
	Age 4–7 years: energy 685 kJ—10% RDI; protein 5.4 g—22% RDI
	Age 8–11 years: energy 685 kJ—10% RDI; protein 5.4 g—14% RDI

Ingredients

Makes 2 serves

1/2 cup milk

1 teaspoon sugar

1 teaspoon drinking chocolate powder

1 egg, lightly beaten

1/2 very ripe pear, cored, peeled and mashed

Method

- Warm the milk in the top of a double boiler over simmering water.
- Add the sugar and drinking chocolate powder.
- Reduce heat and stir in the beaten egg.
- Keep stirring over a gentle heat until the custard thickens (10–20 minutes).
- Pour over the mashed pear.

Nutritional analysis per serve	Age 1–3 years: energy 530 kJ—10% RDI; protein 6 g—35% RDI
	Age 4–7 years: energy 530 kJ— 6% RDI; protein 6 g—24% RDI
	Age 8–11 years: energy 530 kJ— 6% RDI; protein 6 g—16% RDI

Ingredients

Makes approximately:
4 serves for 1–3 year olds
3 serves for 4–7 year olds
2 serves for 8–11 year olds

180 g pieces chicken maryland, skinless

40 g onion, sliced

1 teaspoon soy sauce

50 g canned apricots, drained

Method

- Cut each maryland at the joint and place into a casserole dish.
- Sprinkle with sliced onion and soy sauce.
- Puree or mash apricots and pour over chicken, cover and cook at 180°C for $1^1/_2$ hours.

Nutritional analysis per serve

Age 1–3 years: energy 290 kJ—5% RDI; protein 9 g—50% RDI
Age 4–7 years: energy 390 kJ—5% RDI; protein 11 g—45% RDI
Age 8–11 years: energy 585 kJ—7% RDI; protein 17 g—45% RDI

Ingredients

Makes approximately:
- 4 serves for 1–3 year olds
- 3 serves for 4–7 year olds
- 2 serves for 8–11 year olds

1 small onion, finely chopped

30 g butter

3 tablespoons flour

1 cup milk

1 x 180 g can tuna in springwater

1 x 130 g can creamed corn

1 cup cooked rice

1–2 teaspoons chopped fresh parsley

1 tablespoon lemon juice

Method

- Place onion and butter in a medium saucepan and cook over medium heat until softened.
- Stir in flour, blending well.
- Drain tuna, reserving liquid. Make up liquid with 1/2 cup water.
- Add to flour and onion and stir well.
- Stir in milk.
- Cook over medium heat for 2–3 minutes, stirring constantly.
- Add corn, tuna, rice and parsley.
- Mix thoroughly and cook a further 3 minutes, stirring constantly.
- Serve drizzled with lemon juice and season to taste with freshly ground pepper.

Nutritional analysis per serve

Age 1–3 years: energy 775 kJ—13% RDI; protein 12 g—65% RDI
Age 4–7 years: energy 1030 kJ—13% RDI; protein 16 g—65% RDI
Age 8–11 years: energy 1550 kJ—13% RDI; protein 16 g—42% RDI

Ingredients

Makes approximately:
8 serves for 1–3 year olds
6 serves for 4–7 year olds
4 serves for 8–11 year olds

1 x 220 g can salmon or tuna, drained

juice of 1 lemon

1 cup dry breadcrumbs

$^3/_4$ cup white sauce (see below)

250 g tomatoes, peeled and sliced

1 cup grated mozzarella cheese

White sauce

3 teaspoons monounsaturated margarine

2 teaspoons white flour

$^3/_4$ cup milk

Method

- To make sauce, melt margarine then add flour, mixing well to a smooth paste to make a roux. Cool. Bring milk to the boil then allow to cool for a few minutes. Gradually pour milk into the roux, mixing well with a wooden spoon to avoid lumps. If lumps form, pass through a fine strainer. Makes $^3/_4$ cup.
- Mash fish, remove any bones.
- Place fish and lemon juice in a buttered ovenproof dish. Cover with half the breadcrumbs, the white sauce and a layer of tomatoes.
- Cover with remaining breadcrumbs, top with cheese and bake in a moderate oven for 20 minutes.

Nutritional analysis per serve

Age 1–3 years: energy 740 kJ—12% RDI; protein 13 g—70% RDI
Age 4–7 years: energy 980 kJ—12% RDI; protein 17 g—70% RDI
Age 8–11 years: energy 1475 kJ—17% RDI; protein 27 g—70% RDI

A great way to add kilojoules and protein to soups and vegetable casseroles.

Ingredients

Makes approximately 5 serves

1 tablespoon butter

1 egg

3 tablespoons flour

salt to taste (omit for toddlers and young children)

Method

- Beat the butter well until it becomes light and frothy.
- Add the lightly beaten egg and flour and beat well with a spoon.
- Spoon the dough into boiling soup and cook until tender—this takes only a few minutes.

Nutritional analysis per serve	Age 1–3 years: energy 500 kJ—8% RDI; protein 3 g—17% RDI
	Age 4–7 years: energy 500 kJ—6% RDI; protein 3 g—12% RDI
	Age 8–11 years: energy 500 kJ—6% RDI; protein 3 g— 8% RDI

A very fast way to add protein and kilojoules to soups and vegetable casseroles.

Ingredients

Makes 5 serves

1 egg

1 tablespoon milk

$1\frac{1}{2}$ tablespoons flour

salt to taste (omit for toddlers and young children)

Method

- Beat the eggs well.
- Stir in the milk, flour and salt, and mix well.
- Pour into boiling soup.
- Cook for a minute or two before serving.

Nutritional analysis per serve	Age 1–3 years: energy 130 kJ—2% RDI; protein 2 g—10% RDI
	Age 4–7 years: energy 130 kJ—2% RDI; protein 2 g— 8% RDI
	Age 8–11 years: energy 130 kJ—2% RDI; protein 2 g— 5% RDI

Children will love these. For young children, bake on a greased tray instead of frying.

Ingredients

Makes approximately:
8 serves for 1–3 year olds
6 serves for 4–7 year olds
4 serves for 8–11 year olds

6 small potatoes, raw

40 g self-raising flour

3 teaspoons whole milk

40 g butter

45 g egg

salt to taste (omit for toddlers and young children)

Method

- Wash and peel the potatoes.
- Grate them very finely, strain off liquid.
- Place the grated potatoes in a dish, add salt and flour.
- Mix in milk with a spoon until a batter is formed.
- In a frying pan, heat the butter until hot, scoop the batter with a spoon and fry small pancakes on both sides until golden brown.

Nutritional analysis per serve
Age 1–3 years: energy 415 kJ— 7% RDI; protein 3 g—17% RDI
Age 4–7 years: energy 555 kJ— 7% RDI; protein 4 g—15% RDI
Age 8–11 years: energy 840 kJ—10% RDI; protein 6 g—15% RDI

Cut into quarters before serving for toddlers.

Ingredients

Makes 1 serve

3 tablespoons tomato pasta sauce

35 g minced beef

1 teaspoon parsley

1 tablespoon mushroom, chopped and fried

30 g white crumpet, toasted

Method

- Stir-fry minced beef in a little oil.
- Toast crumpet lightly.
- Spread with tomato sauce.
- Top with minced beef and mushrooms and sprinkle with parsley.
- Sprinkle lightly with cheese.
- Grill for a few minutes until cheese is golden.

Nutritional analysis per serve

Age 1–3 years: energy 655 kJ—10% RDI; protein 10 g—56% RDI
Age 4–7 years: energy 655 kJ— 8% RDI; protein 10 g—40% RDI
Age 8–11 years: energy 655 kJ— 8% RDI; protein 10 g—25% RDI

Cut into quarters before serving for toddlers.

Ingredients

Makes 1 serve

50 g spinach, chopped and cooked

50 g ricotta cheese

30 g mozzarella cheese

30 g white crumpet, toasted

Method

- Mix spinach and ricotta cheese together.
- Toast crumpet lightly.
- Top with spinach and ricotta mixture.
- Sprinkle lightly with mozzarella cheese.
- Grill until cheese is golden.

Nutritional analysis per serve	Age 1–3 years: energy 1000 kJ—16% RDI; protein 16 g—88% RDI
	Age 4–7 years: energy 1000 kJ—12% RDI; protein 16 g—67% RDI
	Age 8–11 years: energy 1000 kJ—11% RDI; protein 16 g—42% RDI

Ingredients

Makes 1 serve

1 egg

4 tablespoons whole milk

5 g spring onion

15 g bacon, middle, fat trimmed or lean ham

10 g margarine

Method

- Chop bacon or ham and fry lightly in margarine.
- Break the eggs into the pan with the bacon.
- Add the milk.
- Mix carefully as they set.
- Finally, add the finely chopped spring onions.
- Toss lightly and serve.

Nutritional analysis per serve	Age 1–3 years: energy 935 kJ—15% RDI; protein 13 g—74% RDI Age 4–7 years: energy 935 kJ—11% RDI; protein 13 g—54% RDI Age 8–11 years: energy 935 kJ—11% RDI; protein 13 g—34% RDI

2

Vitamin A against infection

Vitamin A (properly known as retinol) plays a vital role in protecting children against respiratory and other infections. It is so important for a healthy immune system that it has earned itself the name of the 'anti-infection' vitamin. It manages to strengthen children's immunity by being in a number of places at once, supervising chemical reactions that improve children's resistance to microbes. Vitamin A plays a particularly important role in preventing skin diseases, and respiratory infections in children.

Vitamin A is vital for the healthy formation of epithelial cells, which together form a physical barrier against the entry of infectious microbes into children's bodies. Epithelial cells cover surfaces on the outside as well as on the inside of the body. They are present in the lungs, the inner ear, the nose, the cornea of the eye and many other areas. For example, the epithelial cells in the lungs and bronchi help to guard against respiratory infections. The epithelial cells secrete a mucus that offers additional protection against the entry of bugs into living cells. The ability of these cells to guard against foreign invaders depends on adequate levels of vitamin A, which strengthens their structural integrity.

Studies show that even a mild deficiency of vitamin A in children places them at higher risk of catching respiratory infections. A study looking at the rates of respiratory infections in children found that children with a mild vitamin A deficiency were ill more often than children whose vitamin A levels were normal, or were returning to normal via supplementation. Other studies looking at supplementing vitamin A in children found that it boosted the levels of a natural substance called lactoferrin in tears. Lactoferrin helps to guard against infections caused by bacteria, viruses and fungi, which can enter children's eyes in large numbers when children rub their eyes, for example.

A Californian study that looked at vitamin A levels in children with measles found that half the children with measles were deficient in vitamin A. The children who were deficient in vitamin A had a longer duration of illness and more severe complications, including pneumonia. The risk of developing serious respiratory complications as a result of vitamin A deficiency during measles is now well recognised by the Australian College of Paediatrics, which recommends vitamin A injections for children with measles who are low in the vitamin. Lack of vitamin A allows viral infections to gain a stronger foothold, leading to more severe symptoms.

Vitamin A regulates gene expression

Recent research has shown that vitamin A influences the expression of genes that are vital to a robust immune system. In other words, it regulates the making of some components of the immune system from scratch. The presence or absence of vitamin A influences commands at the genetic level, at the control centre for protein production. Its function at the genetic level can be likened to decision making at army headquarters where the general decides what troops and how many to send out to stage a defence against an invading force. Low levels of vitamin A can make the attack less effective, due to insufficient or less efficient white blood cells.

Vitamin A is needed for the immune system's ability to generate normal fighter cells in adequate numbers. These fighter cells include macrophages, which gobble up bacteria and other foreign debris, neutrophils, and the B and T cells of the adaptive immune system. Vitamin A deficiency reduces the number of natural killer cells which, you may recall, are important in the first-line defence against viruses. Vitamin A also stimulates the immune system to act swiftly against bacteria.

Vitamin A enhances the production of antibodies. Antibodies are proteins that latch on to foreign structures on microbes in order to destroy them. This is rather like throwing a net to catch and immobilise an opponent. Vitamin A improves the speed at which the body makes antibodies by using specific types of fighter cells called T-helper cells and phagocytes. This is particularly important to fight bacterial infections. It also helps the immune system's ability to heal infected tissues and to increase resistance to further infection.

Infection reduces body stores of vitamin A

Acute infection has been shown to deplete body stores of vitamin A. As a result, some scientists question whether the recommended daily intake (RDI) for vitamin A is sufficient for children who are ill. The RDI is set at a level that will prevent nutrient deficiency in healthy children. Studies are under way to determine the optimal amount for children during illness. Don't be tempted to self-prescribe a vitamin A supplement for your child as these can be toxic if taken in high doses or over a long period of time. You'll find more information on vitamin A supplements in Chapter 9.

What is the most prudent thing to do meanwhile? Well, if you have a child who suffers from recurrent respiratory or other infections don't hesitate to consider the possibility of vitamin A deficiency. If you want to be sure, take your child to a doctor and ask for a blood test that will show your child's vitamin A level. If the level is too low, your doctor may decide to give your child a vitamin A injection. Then you must give attention to your child's diet as this is the only long-term measure to prevent vitamin A deficiency from occurring again in the future.

Read on to find out how to make sure your child gets sufficient amounts of vitamin A from the diet.

Children's needs for vitamin A

Children need more vitamin A per kilogram weight than adults. For toddlers the daily recommended intake is 300 micrograms. For young children aged 4–7 years the RDI increases to 350 micrograms, and for older children aged 8–11 years it is 500 micrograms. Remember that children eat much less than adults and so their diet must be relatively higher in vitamin A. Putting it simply, children's diets must contain more vitamin A per mouthful.

Sources of vitamin A

The richest source of vitamin A is liver, but it is not necessary to include liver as part of children's diets unless it is well liked—there are other good sources. Dairy products, eggs and oily fish (e.g. salmon, mackerel, sardines) are all very good sources of vitamin A.

If you like to include liver in your child's diet, bear in mind that it is very rich in vitamin A and if given too often can cause a build up of vitamin A to toxic levels. For example, 10 grams of cooked liver has 3540 micrograms retinol—that's ten times the RDI for young children. So avoid large serves, particularly for small children.

Provitamin A

Provitamin A refers to the carotenoids, a family of plant molecules that can be turned into fully active vitamin A once inside the body. Children who eat a diet rich in carotenoids make some of their vitamin A in this way. But not all carotenoids are well absorbed and research shows that the colour of vegetables and fruits is a good guide. Yellow-coloured vegetables contain beta carotene which is well absorbed. (More on beta carotene on p. 185–6.) Excellent sources of beta carotene are pumpkin, carrots, yellow squash, sweet potato, tomatoes and—in the fruits—mango, papaya, rockmelon, persimmon and apricots.

Remember that once picked, fruits and foods that are dried in, or exposed to, sunlight lose most of their vitamin A. Cooking food at lower temperatures minimises the loss of vitamin A, so steaming and boiling are the methods of choice in preference to baking or frying.

It's easy to make sure children have sufficient amounts of vitamin A every day. Simply pick a combination of foods from Table 2.1.

Table 2.1

Vitamin A content of foods

Food	Portion	Amount (mcg RE*)
Vegetables (cooked)		
Cabbage	40 g	37
Carrot	1/4 cup	612
Pumpkin	1/4 cup	248
Spinach, English	1/4 cup	130
Squash, button	1/4 cup	28
Sweet potato	1/4 cup	423
Tomato	45 g	26
Fruit (raw)		
Apricot	small	112
Mango	1/2 of fruit	400
Pawpaw	1/4 cup	60
Rockmelon/cantaloupe	1/2 cup	118
Others		
Butter, regular	1 tsp	51
Cheese, cheddar (mild, tasty, vintage)	30 g	117
Cheese, ricotta	30 g	33
Egg, whole, raw	45 g	72
Margarine	1 tsp	46
Milk, fluid, whole	100 ml	49

* RE = retinol equivalents. RDI for vitamin A for children 1–3 years is 300 mcg RE; for children 4–7 years 350 mcg RE; and for children 8–11 years 500 mcg RE.

Source: FoodWorks Professional Edition, Copyright 1998–2000 Xyris Software.

This soup is extremely rich in beta carotene which is converted to vitamin A once inside the body.

Ingredients

Makes approximately 8 serves

1 tablespoon butter

1 small onion, finely chopped

2 cups chicken stock

500 g carrots, washed, scrubbed and chopped

1 cup orange juice

chopped parsley to garnish (omit for very young children)

Method

- Melt butter and cook onion until transparent.
- Add carrots and toss for one minute.
- Add chicken stock and simmer for 10 minutes.
- Place mixture in a blender and blend till smooth.
- Return soup to saucepan and add orange juice.
- Heat without boiling.
- Garnish with chopped parsley.

Nutritional analysis per serve	*Vitamin A* Age 1–3 years: 1095 mcg—365% RDI Age 4–7 years: 1095 mcg—315% RDI Age 8–11 years: 1095 mcg—220% RDI

Ingredients

Makes approximately 8 serves

140 g cauliflower florets

3 cups chicken stock

1 sprig parsley (omit for very young children)

2/3 cup evaporated fat-reduced milk, unsweetened

1 tablespoon butter

1/2 cup grated cheddar cheese

Method

- Cook cauliflower in boiling stock until tender.
- Cool slightly.
- Puree cauliflower mixture in a blender, then return to saucepan, stir well.
- Add butter, evaporated fat-reduced milk and cheese.
- Simmer very gently over low heat. Do not boil.
- Serve sprinkled with finely chopped parsley.

Nutritional analysis per serve

Vitamin A
Age 1–3 years: 60 mcg—20% RDI
Age 4–7 years: 60 mcg—17% RDI
Age 8–11 years: 60 mcg—12% RDI

Ingredients

Makes approximately 1 serve

3 tablespoons smooth ricotta cheese

1 egg, lightly beaten

2 tablespoons flaked, cooked or canned tuna

Method

- Preheat oven to 180°C.
- Beat cheese and egg well in a small mixing bowl.
- Add tuna and mix well.
- Pour mixture into a baking mould and bake at 180°C for 25–30 minutes until set in the centre.
- Stand for 5 minutes.
- Turn out and serve with toast or salad.

Nutritional analysis per serve

Vitamin A
Age 1–3 years: 85 mcg—30% RDI
Age 4–7 years: 85 mcg—25% RDI
Age 8–11 years: 85 mcg—15% RDI

Mango is a great source of vitamin A.

Ingredients

Makes approximately:
6 serves for 1–3 year olds
5 serves for 4–7 year olds
4 serves for 8–11 year olds

400 g bream fillets

1 stick celery, sliced

1 mango, peeled and sliced

1/2 cup water

juice of 1/2 lemon

2 tablespoons cornflour

Method

- Cut fish into 4–6 pieces.
- Place in a medium glass casserole dish.
- Top with celery and mango, pour water and orange juice over.
- Cover container with aluminium foil and cook at 200°C for 20 minutes.
- Remove fish, celery and mango from liquid.
- Blend cornflour with a little water to dissolve.
- Add to liquid and stir well.
- Reheat, stirring until thickened.
- Pour sauce over fish.

Nutritional analysis per serve

Vitamin A
Age 1–3 years: 140 mcg—45% RDI
Age 4–7 years: 170 mcg—50% RDI
Age 8–11 years: 215 mcg—45% RDI

A small amount of paté goes a long way, so avoid serving more than the recommended serve.

Ingredients

Makes approximately 5 serves

3 teaspoons monounsaturated margarine

10 g rindless bacon, chopped

20 g onion, finely chopped

1 g garlic, finely sliced

grated nutmeg

ground black pepper

60 g chicken livers, trimmed and chopped

1 teaspoon chopped fresh coriander or parsley

3 ml brandy

salt to taste (omit for toddlers and young children)

Method

- Put the magarine, bacon, onion, garlic, nutmeg and pepper in a large, heavy-based frying pan.
- Cook over medium heat for 5 minutes, stirring frequently.
- Add the livers and salt. Cook, stirring frequently, for 5–10 minutes, until all the liver has changed colour.
- Stir in the coriander and brandy. Cool slightly.
- Mix in a food processor to a smooth texture. Put into several small bowls or one large bowl and refrigerate until set.
- Serve spread on fingers of toast or rusks.

Nutritional analysis per serve	*Vitamin A* Age 1–3 years: 770 mcg—250% RDI Age 4–7 years: 770 mcg—220% RDI Age 8–11 years: 770 mcg—155% RDI

Ingredients

Makes approximately
5 serves for 1–3 year olds
4 serves for 4–7 year olds
3 serves for 8–11 year olds

2/3 cup cooked brown lentils

1/4 cup mashed potato

1/2 medium sweet potato

2 tablespoons sesame seeds

1 tablespoon ground sunflower seeds

2 tablespoons grated carrot

1/4 small onion, grated

1/4 cup ricotta cheese

splash of soy sauce to taste

fresh tomato sauce

Method

- Combine all ingredients and mix well.
- Shape into patties and place on greased oven tray.
- Bake at 200°C for approximately 20 minutes.
- Serve with fresh tomato sauce.

Nutritional analysis per serve

Vitamin A
Age 1–3 years: 185 mcg—60% RDI
Age 4–7 years: 230 mcg—65% RDI
Age 8–11 years: 310 mcg—60% RDI

This is another soup rich in beta carotene.

Ingredients

Makes approximately 8 serves

1 tablespoon olive oil

1 small onion, chopped

400 ml chicken stock

300 g pumpkin, peeled and cut into 5-cm pieces

400 ml milk, hot

1/4 teaspoon nutmeg

salt and pepper to taste

1 teaspoon parsley, chopped (omit for very young children)

Method

- Heat oil, sauté onion until soft.
- Add chicken stock and bring to boil.
- Add pumpkin pieces and simmer until soft (10–15 minutes).
- Add hot milk, nutmeg, salt and pepper.
- Heat through until almost boiling.
- Immediately before serving, sprinkle with parsley.

Nutritional analysis per serve

Vitamin A
Age 1–3 years: 235 mcg—78% RDI
Age 4–7 years: 235 mcg—80% RDI
Age 8–11 years: 235 mcg—55% RDI

Ingredients

Makes approximately 4 serves

100 g skinless chicken

100 g pumpkin

3/4 cup chicken stock

2 teaspoons cornflour

1 tablespoon toasted sesame seeds

Method

- Chop chicken and pumpkin into 2-cm pieces.
- Place in a medium saucepan.
- Pour over 1/2 cup stock.
- Cover and simmer over a low heat for 15 minutes until pumpkin is soft. Cool.
- Puree pumpkin and chicken mixture.
- Blend cornflour in remaining stock until dissolved, add to pumpkin mixture, stir well.
- Warm sauce on low heat for 4–5 minutes, stirring several times.
- Serve over pasta of your choice and top with toasted sesame seeds.

Nutritional analysis per serve

Vitamin A
Age 1–3 years: 130 mcg—45% RDI
Age 4–7 years: 130 mcg—35% RDI
Age 8–11 years: 130 mcg—25% RDI

Ingredients

Makes approximately 4 serves

2 tablespoons olive oil

1 1/2 cups chopped onion

3 cups peeled, diced eggplant

1/2 cup chopped red capsicum

1/2 cup peeled, chopped carrot

3 cloves garlic, peeled

2 cups water

salt and ground black pepper to taste (omit for toddlers and young children)

Method

- In a large skillet with a lid, heat oil over medium-high heat.
- Add onion and cook, stirring often, until lightly browned, about 5 minutes.
- Add eggplant and cook, stirring often until browned, about 5 minutes.
- Add capsicum, carrot, garlic and water.
- Bring to boil, reduce heat, cover; simmer for 30 minutes or until vegetables are soft.
- Season with salt and pepper.
- Transfer sauce to a food processor or blender and puree.
- Serve right away over some pasta.

Nutritional analysis per serve

Vitamin A
Age 1–3 years: 330 mcg—110% RDI
Age 4–7 years: 330 mcg— 95% RDI
Age 8–11 years: 330 mcg— 65% RDI

Ingredients

Makes approximately 6 serves

450 g canned pie apricots

3–4 tablespoons water

1/2 cup plain flour

1/2 cup instant raw oats

1/4 cup butter or monounsaturated margarine

1/4 cup sugar

Method

- Put the fruit into an ovenproof dish.
- Add water.
- Add sugar to sweeten.
- Cook gently in the oven for 10–15 minutes.
- Sieve the flour.
- Add instant oats and mix.
- Rub in the butter or margarine, add the sugar and mix.
- Sprinkle over the top of the fruit.
- Bake in the centre of a moderate oven at 180°C for 25–30 minutes.

Nutritional analysis per serve

Vitamin A
Age 1–3 years: 275 mcg—90% RDI
Age 4–7 years: 275 mcg—80% RDI
Age 8–11 years: 275 mcg—55% RDI

Ingredients

Makes approximately:
6 serves for 1–3 year olds
5 serves for 4–7 year olds
4 serves for 8–11 year olds

325 g chicken thigh fillets
1½ tablespoons canola oil
1 onion, cut into rings
60 g baby sweet corn, cut into quarters
60 g carrots, sliced thinly and cut into shapes with a tiny biscuit cutter
90 g broccoli, cut into small florets
90 g bean sprouts
30 g red capsicum, cored, deseeded and cut into strips
1 spring onion, finely chopped
pinch of black pepper

Sweet and sour sauce

150 ml vegetable stock
½ tablespoon cornflour blended with 1 tablespoon cold water
1 teaspoon brown sugar
1 tablespoon soy sauce

Method

- Cut chicken fillets into strips.
- In a wok, stir-fry chicken in oil until golden.
- Add the onion and sauté until softened.
- Add sweet corn, carrots and broccoli, and stir-fry for 2 minutes.
- Add the bean sprouts, red capsicum and spring onions, and stir-fry for a further 2 minutes.
- Season with a little black pepper.
- To make sauce, blend the vegetable stock with the cornflour paste in a small pan.
- Mix in the brown sugar and soy sauce.
- Over a high heat, bring to boil and simmer for about 2 minutes, until sauce thickens.
- Toss the hot vegetables in the sauce, and heat through in the wok.

Nutritional analysis per serve

Vitamin A
Age 1–3 years: 195 mcg—65% RDI
Age 4–7 years: 235 mcg—65% RDI
Age 8–11 years: 290 mcg—58% RDI

3

Iron for strong immunity

Many studies show the importance of iron to a healthy immune system. Studies with infants show that anaemic infants suffer more infections than infants with adequate iron stores. A Chicago study found that supplementation of iron to children suffering frequent respiratory infections significantly lowered the incidence of infections. The same study reported that iron supplementation of children who were well nourished had no significant effect. This underlines the importance of iron supplementation for children who are deficient in iron but shows no further benefits for children with normal levels of iron. It also points to iron's important role in protecting children against infection.

Another study looked at fortifying cow's milk with iron, to see whether this form of iron supplementation was helpful in preventing respiratory infections. The results showed that only 9% of the children who drank iron-fortified milk succumbed to respiratory infections compared with 76% of the children who were not supplemented with iron.

Iron deficiency has the following effects on the immune system:

- reduces the ability of the immune system to fight bacteria;
- slows down the transformation of fighter cells from being dormant to being primed and ready to attack foreign microbes;
- slows down cellular defences in general;
- possibly slows down the activities of antioxidant enzymes.

In addition, some research implies that dietary iron—just like the metal in the real world—is used in the manufacture of ammunition, except that dietary iron is used against bacteria and other harmful pathogens. The iron helps to make small protein structures called *antibodies*. Antibodies are 'fired' against the enemy ranks, which in our scenario are foreign cellular structures. Without sufficient iron the production of antibodies cannot take place, or takes place at a very slow rate. Children deficient in iron are more likely to have an immune system that is like a poorly equipped army—ready to fight but with little ammunition to raise the attack.

Increased iron needs in childhood

Growing requires a lot of work. The period of childhood growth is a very busy time for the body; on top of staying healthy, it must also build and strengthen itself. The bone matrix and muscle fibres must be made anew and then strengthened. The amount of blood must keep up with the child's growing body and so all the cells and blood particles are made at a faster rate. Some will replace the old, used cells and some will be new additions to meet the extra needs of the growing body. Hence it is little wonder that, in times of rapid growth, the need for iron is much greater.

Iron is directed into red blood cells to make them efficient at carrying oxygen in the blood. Without sufficient iron the red blood cells are unable to carry enough oxygen, and oxygen is essential for cellular metabolism, or the generation of energy from the food we eat. So every red blood cell requires a specific, small but essential amount of iron. And there are lots of red blood cells to be made.

Lack of iron results in red blood cells that don't deliver an adequate supply of oxygen to the cells in the body. The result is a tired and listless child who is also more likely to fall victim to infections.

Do children lack iron in their diets?

Iron received special attention during the setting up of the Australian Dietary Guidelines for children. There is a separate dietary guideline for iron alone which I quote here: 'Eat foods containing iron.' It reminds us to look more closely at the iron content of children's diets because children are more vulnerable to iron deficiency.

Surveys on iron levels in children are lacking. The Australian National Nutrition Survey (1995) did not find low intakes of iron in children. However iron intake can vary greatly from day to day and a minimum of three days gives a more representative iron intake. Perhaps more importantly, the survey did not differentiate between haem and non-haem iron intakes—we will look at these in the following sections.

Children at risk of iron deficiency

In 1994 I had the opportunity to coordinate a study that looked at the amount of iron in the diets of toddlers living in the central Sydney area. The study was undertaken by the Central Sydney

Health Area together with the Division of General Practice. Briefly, the study involved:

- taking a sample of the children's blood to test their iron levels;
- obtaining a food diary kept by the children's parents/carers who weighed and recorded the children's usual diet for three days;
- analysing the food diary for the amount of iron and other nutrients in the children's diets;
- comparing the children's blood iron levels with the amount of iron in their diets.

We found that children who were low in iron consumed on average slightly less total iron than children who had adequate iron levels—the difference was not significant. It became clear that children who loved milk and other dairy products were eating less iron-rich food, in particular less food rich in haem iron, such as meat, and this group of children was much more likely to be iron-deficient as shown by the blood tests. I took three important messages from this study regarding iron nutrition in children:

1. Some young children in urban Sydney suffer from iron deficiency. Two recent Australian studies have also found that 30% of children under the age of two had iron deficiency.
2. Although important for children's health, milk and dairy products must be limited to a recommended allowance if they are not to replace iron-rich foods in the diet.
3. A lack of red meat in children's diets makes them more susceptible to iron deficiency unless food substitutes rich in haem iron become part of their daily diets.

Different types of iron

Iron in the foods that children eat is found in two forms: *haem* iron is found in liver, kidneys and lean red meats, poultry and seafood, while *non-haem* iron is found in legumes, egg yolks, wholemeal breads, wholegrain cereals, green leafy vegetables, nuts and seeds. There is some non-haem iron in muscle proteins but there is no haem iron in plant foods. Haem iron is well absorbed by our bodies, while non-haem iron is absorbed rather poorly. Less than 5% of non-haem iron is absorbed compared with 10–25% of the haem iron in meat muscle. Therefore, although plant sources contain relatively high amounts of non-haem iron, this type of iron is not as well absorbed. Children who rely on non-haem iron foods to supply them with their iron must eat more iron-rich foods than children who eat foods rich in haem iron. To prevent iron deficiency, the diets of these children should include frequent, generous amounts of non-haem rich foods.

We look at vegeterian diets which rely solely on plants to provide children's iron needs in Chapter 7.

The absorption of non-haem iron can be increased by providing vitamin C with meals containing non-haem iron. By including vegetables that are good sources of vitamin C, or offering fruit rich in vitamin C just after the meal, the overall non-haem iron absorption can be increased up to four times. To achieve these benefits the vitamin C and non-haem iron must be consumed at the same meal. Recent research shows that citric acid, which is plentiful in citrus fruit (oranges, grapefruits, lemons), enhances the absorption of iron in addition to vitamin C, so serving citrus fruit or diluted citrus fruit juice will further increase the absorption of non-haem iron.

Good sources of non-haem (less well absorbed) iron: green leafy vegetables, wheat germ, wholegrain cereals, wholemeal breads, nuts, dried peas and beans, lentils, prunes, dates and apricots.

Good sources of haem (well absorbed) iron: liver, lean red meat, lean chicken (thigh meat has more haem iron than breast meat) and fish, particularly dark-fleshed fish (e.g. tuna, salmon).

On the other hand, iron absorption is inhibited by:

- phytates, which make up 1–2% of many cereals, nuts and legumes;
- polyphenols, which are present in tea, cocoa and legumes; and
- soy proteins.

Refined grains are much lower in phytates than wholegrain cereals, but the iron content of wholegrain cereals is higher than that of refined cereals so the higher content of wholegrain cereals compensates for the poorer absorption. In addition, yeast breaks down the structure of phytates and so improves the absorption of iron from baked products such as bread. The addition of vitamin C to a meal containing nuts or legumes (dried beans, lentils, peas) also helps to counteract the inhibiting effect of phytates on iron absorption.

Polyphenols (e.g. tannins in tea and cocoa) reduce the absorption of non-haem iron by half. This can be readily avoided by not serving tea or cocoa drinks to children at mealtimes. Reserve these drinks for between meals or for supper when they are least likely to reduce iron absorption. In addition, calcium in dairy products can markedly reduce iron absorption. Again, not mixing food sources high in calcium and iron in the one meal will prevent this. Soy milk is not a good drink to have with a meal either because it has proteins that bind iron, making it more difficult for the iron to be absorbed.

So, to improve iron absorption from a meal:

- Offer diluted fruit juice, or citrus fruit, with or after meals.
- Include vegetables rich in vitamin C as part of a meal.
- Avoid serving tea, cola, cocoa or milk with a meal that is rich in iron.

Breakfast cereals

The fortification of breakfast cereals with iron has helped to put more iron into children's diets, but it is important to realise that breakfast cereals are fortified with iron that is rather poorly absorbed. And while its absorption can be increased by including fruit rich in vitamin C with breakfast, cereals are often served with milk or soy milk, both of which will inhibit the amount of iron absorbed. Yes, breakfast cereal helps to increase the iron content of children's diets, but the question remains: how much of it is absorbed? We need to get away from the figures on the breakfast cereal box and think of how much iron actually gets inside the child's body. There's no need to exclude breakfast cereals from your child's diet, but don't consider them a major source of iron (easily done when looking at the figures on the box).

If your children won't eat meat

This section applies mainly to young children as the reasons for older children not eating meat were discussed in Chapter 1. First of all, it is important to discover why young children won't eat meat. The most common reasons are:

- They fill up on large quantities of milk, which is much easier to consume—who would want to chew when they can simply swallow?
- They don't like, or are not used to, the texture of meat—you must persevere here.
- They don't like the taste—there are many ways to cook meat.
- They don't like the thought of killing animals.

Young children will generally go for the easier and tastier option, while parents may be too busy to notice how much milk their child drinks. Meat takes longer to feed to a child, and it takes some time for the child to get used to it and to learn to like and accept it. But dairy food is no substitute for meat.

Try chicken thigh meat if red meat is a 'no go' to start with. Include very small pieces of red meat in a casserole. Then build up to spaghetti bolognaise and so on. The actual food choices will depend to some extent on your child's age and preferences, but remember that your goal is to include more haem iron in your child's diet, so do persevere. Browse through the recipe section to find other ideas to substitute for red meat dishes as well as some easier-to-like red meat dishes for children of different ages.

Supplements

Despite the role that iron plays in preventing infections, a number of studies in children found that too much iron may actually make things worse. Too much iron in the blood appears to change its chemistry in favour of the bugs. Elevated levels of free iron in the blood become food for bacteria and they start to multiply faster. This is why it pays to be cautious with iron supplements.

Don't give iron supplements to children until you are sure they have low blood levels of iron. Ask your doctor to check this out and give a supplement only if your doctor thinks it is appropriate. Iron levels in the blood fall naturally after an infection so don't forget to mention to your doctor if your child has been ill. Do return for a recheck of your child's iron levels as indicated by your doctor. Remember, large doses of iron are hazardous for children so don't ever be tempted to give your child an iron supplement meant for adults.

Some reports indicate that iron supplements should be avoided during acute infections, particularly in young children, so if your child takes an iron supplement it may be wise to stop the

Table 3.1

Iron content of foods

Food	**Portion**	**Amount (mg)***
Bread and Cereals (less well absorbed)		
Bread, white	24 g	0.3
Bread, wholemeal	24 g	0.5
Oats	1/2 cup	0.7
Breakfast cereal	28 g	2.4
Pearl barley	1/2 cup	1.0
Rice, white	1/2 cup	0.3
Rice, brown	1/2 cup	0.5
Wheat germ	1 tbsp	0.6
Fruit and Vegetables (less well absorbed)		
Avocado, raw	40 g	0.3
Baked beans	1/4 cup	1.1
Broccoli, cooked	45 g	0.5
Brussels sprouts	1/4 cup	0.6
Chickpeas	1/4 cup	2.8
Lentils	1/4 cup	0.9
Peas	1/4 cup	0.5
Prunes	40 g	0.5
Prunes, stewed	40 g	0.1
Pumpkin, boiled	1/4 cup	0.3
Raisins	25 g	1.1
Soybeans	1/4 cup	0.9
Spinach, English, cooked	1/4 cup	1.1
Meat and Alternatives (raw)		
(well absorbed)		
Beef	45 g	1.0
Chicken, breast	45 g	0.3
Chicken, thigh	45 g	0.5
Fish	45 g	0.3
Lamb	45 g	0.8
Pork	45 g	0.4
Veal	45 g	0.7
(less well absorbed)		
Bean curd (tofu)	40 g	3.2
Cashew	15 g	0.8
Egg	45 g	0.7
Molasses	1 tsp	0.3
Pumpkin seeds	15 g	1.5
Sunflower seeds	15 g	0.7
Tahini, sesame butter	15 g	0.8
Walnut	15 g	0.4

* RDI for all children is 6–8 mg daily.
Source: FoodWorks Professional Edition, Copyright 1998–2000 Xyris Software.

supplement during illness and wait until your child is better before restarting it. With iron, as with all other nutrients, a nutritional balance is the key and food sources are the best and safest way to get your child's nutrient levels back to normal.

Table 3.1 gives the iron content of various foods.

Dark-fleshed fish like tuna is higher in iron than white fish.

Ingredients

Makes approximately 5 serves

220 g canned tuna (salt-reduced)

1 tablespoon mayonnaise

1 teaspoon fresh lemon juice

1 teaspoon chopped fresh parsley (omit for very young children)

1/2 teaspoon tomato sauce

1/2 teaspoon Worcestershire sauce

1 teaspoon gelatine dissolved in 1 tablespoon boiling water

Method

- Combine all ingredients in a small bowl.
- Refrigerate until set.
- Serve on crackers with salad vegetables, or as a sandwich filling.

Nutritional analysis per serve *Iron*
For children all ages: 0.5 mg—8% RDI

Ingredients

Makes approximately:
4 serves for 1–3 year olds
2 serves for older children

110 g tinned sardines, drained on paper towel and mashed

1 small apple, peeled, cored, grated

1 teaspoon lemon juice

4 slices wholemeal bread

1/2 cup cheddar cheese

Method

- Toast bread.
- Mix sardines, apple and lemon juice together and pile mixture onto toast.
- Grill until lightly brown.
- Sprinkle with cheese.

Nutritional analysis per serve

Iron
Age 1–3 years: 1.3 mg—20% RDI
Age 4–7 years: 2.6 mg—35% RDI
Age 8–11 years: 2.6 mg—35% RDI

Ingredients

Makes approximately:
8 serves for 1–3 year olds
6 serves for 4–7 year olds
5 serves for 8–11 year olds

500 g finely minced lean beef

1 onion, finely chopped

1 carrot, chopped

1 egg, beaten

1 teaspoon vegemite

1 tablespoon tomato sauce

1 tablespoon fruit chutney

ground black pepper

Method

- Preheat oven to 180°C.
- Combine all ingredients in a bowl and mix thoroughly.
- Spoon the mixture into a 1 kg loaf tin lined with greaseproof paper or baking powder.
- Bake for an hour or until cooked.

Nutritional analysis per serve

Iron
Age 1–3 years: 1.8 mg—25% RDI
Age 4–7 years: 2.3 mg—33% RDI
Age 8–11 years: 2.8 mg—40% RDI

For children over the age of four, you may prefer to use taco shells instead of lavash bread.

Ingredients

Makes approximately:
8 serves for 1–3 year olds
6 serves for older children

500 g topside mince

2 teaspoons olive oil

1 packet tomato soup mix

1/2 teaspoon chilli powder (optional)

1 cup water

1 cup red kidney beans, drained

4 'sheets' lavash bread

1/2 cup thick plain yoghurt

1/2 cup cheddar cheese, grated

Method

- Brown mince in oil.
- Add soup mix, chilli powder, water and beans.
- Simmer for 10 minutes.
- Divide mixture evenly between lavash bread, roll up and place on ovenproof trays.
- Spoon on yoghurt and sprinkle with grated cheese.
- Bake at 200°C for 15–20 minutes.
- Remove from oven and cut into suitable serving size for children.

Nutritional analysis per serve

Iron
Age 1–3 years: 2.9 mg—40% RDI
Age 4–7 years: 3.9 mg—56% RDI
Age 8–11 years: 3.9 mg—56% RDI

Ingredients

Makes approximately:
10 serves for 1–3 year olds
8 serves for 4–7 year olds
5 serves for 8–11 year olds

2 cups flaked fish (fresh, or canned tuna or salmon)

1 cup mashed potato

1 tablespoon chopped parsley (omit for very young children)

1 egg, beaten

wheat germ

Method

- Combine all ingredients except wheat germ.
- Shape mixture into balls and roll in wheat germ.
- Cook in a buttered, ovenproof dish in a moderate oven for 10 minutes, or sauté in oil until brown for older children.

Nutritional analysis per serve

Iron
Age 1–3 years: 0.8 mg—10% RDI
Age 4–7 years: 1.0 mg—15% RDI
Age 8–11 years: 1.6 mg—25% RDI

Broccoli is high in non-haem iron.

Ingredients

Makes approximately 8 serves

2 teaspoons olive oil

1 medium onion, coarsely chopped

4 medium potatoes, coarsely diced

2 cups vegetable stock

1 teaspoon dried thyme

1½ cups milk

3 tablespoons white flour

2 stalks broccoli, cut into large chunks

salt and pepper to taste

½ cup light cream

Method

- In a large pot, heat the olive oil over medium heat.
- Sauté the onion for 2 minutes.
- Add the diced potatoes, the vegetable stock and the thyme.
- Allow the mixture to simmer until the potatoes are tender, about 20 minutes.
- In a blender, blend together the milk and flour.
- Add the broccoli in several additions and process until it is minced.
- Pour the broccoli-milk mixture into the potatoes and onions.
- Bring the soup to a boil.
- Immediately lower the heat and simmer for 10 minutes.
- Add salt and pepper and more thyme to taste.
- Turn off the heat and mix in cream just before serving.

Nutritional analysis per serve	*Iron*
	Age 1–3 years: 0.6 mg—10% RDI
	Age 4–7 years: 0.6 mg—10% RDI
	Age 8–11 years: 0.6 mg—10% RDI

Ingredients

Makes approximately:
12 serves for 1–3 year olds
10 serves for 4–7 year olds
8 serves for 8–11 year olds

1 cup cooked haricot beans

2 carrots

3 potatoes

2 turnips

3 onions

$^1/_2$ bunch celery

chopped parsley (omit for very young children)

3 cups chicken stock

pepper

1 cup grated Swiss cheese

Method

- Prepare haricot beans by soaking in water to cover overnight, then rinsing and boiling them in fresh water until almost cooked, about 1 $^1/_2$–2 hours.
- Prepare vegetables, slice and place in layers with beans and parsley in a flameproof dish with stock.
- Bring to boil, lower heat and gently simmer until vegetables are tender, about 40 minutes.
- Sprinkle with grated cheese and place in oven or under grill until cheese melts.

Nutritional analysis per serve

Iron
Age 1–3 years: 1.6 mg—22% RDI
Age 4–7 years: 1.9 mg—27% RDI
Age 8–11 years: 2.4 mg—34% RDI

Ingredients

Makes approximately 2 serves

2 tablespoons canned tuna in water

1 teaspoon butter or margarine

2 teaspoons flour

100 ml milk

1 teaspoon finely chopped parsley (omit for very young children)

½ hard-boiled egg

2 tablespoons frozen peas (thawed)

1 cup fresh cooked mashed potatoes

Method

- Melt butter in a small saucepan.
- Stir in flour and cook for a few seconds.
- Add milk carefully to avoid lumps.
- Bring to boil, but don't allow to boil over.
- Add parsley and flaked tuna.
- Spread mixture into base of a small casserole dish.
- Slice egg and place in a layer over fish.
- Spread a layer of peas over eggs and lastly a layer of mashed potato.
- Bake at 180°C for 15–20 minutes.
- Cool and serve.

Nutritional analysis per serve

Iron
Age 1–3 years: 1.5 mg—25% RDI
Age 4–7 years: 1.5 mg—25% RDI
Age 8–11 years: 1.5 mg—25% RDI

Use 2 tablespoons ground peanuts or peanut butter for children under 5 years of age.

Ingredients

Makes approximately:
8 serves for 1–3 year olds
6 serves for 4–7 year olds
4 serves for 8–11 year olds

500 g boneless, skinless chicken breast fillets, rinsed and patted dry

1 tablespoon soy sauce

1 tablespoon sweet chilli seasoning

2 tablespoons chopped peanuts

1/2 cup plain dry breadcrumbs

1 lemon, cut in wedges

Method

- Preheat oven to 190°C.
- Cut chicken breasts into finger-length 2-cm wide strips.
- Put chicken strips into a medium bowl.
- Add soy sauce and toss to coat.
- Put sweet chilli seasoning into a small bag, add peanuts or peanut butter and breadcrumbs, shake or rub to mix.
- Transfer chicken to bag with breadcrumbs and shake to coat.
- Press gently to make crumbs adhere to chicken.
- Spread chicken in a single layer on a baking sheet.
- Lightly coat chicken with non-stick cooking spray.
- Bake for 8–10 minutes or until chicken is cooked through and peanut-crumb coating is crisp.
- Serve with lemon wedges.

Nutritional analysis per serve

Iron
Age 1–3 years: 0.7 mg—10% RDI
Age 4–7 years: 0.9 mg—15% RDI
Age 8–11 years: 1.4 mg—20% RDI

4
Zinc's fighting role

In the last 20 years, following the discovery that low body stores of zinc bring about greater susceptibility to infections, zinc has received a good deal of attention among scientists interested in its role in immunity. Researchers are now close to working out the details of how zinc boosts immunity. It is one of the most important nutrients in building immunity and one that is relatively difficult to obtain from the diet, for both adults and children.

Zinc and fighter cells

Without an adequate amount of zinc several types of specialised fighter cells—T cells and B cells as well as natural killer cells—are found to be low in numbers. Zinc, like iron, is important in the production of antibodies and these are in short supply when zinc is deficient. The documented effect of this on a child's health is increased susceptibility to infection and slower wound healing.

Zinc is a vital nutrient for good function of the thymus gland. Studies show that zinc supplementation of people who are low in zinc improves the activity of the thymus gland. The thymus gland is responsible for the production of T cells (T cells because these cells are produced in the thymus.)

The thymus gland is like a factory where the fighter cells are put together and equipped with the right ammunition and communication devices. The ammunition includes antibodies, and communication is possible via small messenger molecules which, when released in the blood by one type of fighter cell, reach other fighter cells by means of cell receptors. *Cell receptors* stick out on the surface of the fighter cells and catch the molecules as they sweep by. Once the receptor locks with a messenger it triggers changes in the fighter cell.

Children who are deficient in zinc develop smaller thymus glands, and the production of T cells slows down. This affects the ability of the immune system to build enough fighters and to orchestrate its defence forces, resulting in a significantly weaker immunity.

Viruses multiplication

Zinc has been shown to prevent the action of viral polypeptides, which can be likened to scissors that cut through the genetic code of a cell. Once a virus gains entry into a healthy cell it tries to merge its own genetic code with that of the cell. In order to do this it 'cuts open' the genetic code and slots in its own genetic features so that its code becomes expressed along with the cell's original DNA. This allows viruses to multiply—they fill up the cell until it is unable to hold on to its contents and bursts.

Zinc seems to be effective in stopping a virus from cutting open a cell's genetic code. When a virus is unable to slot its genetic code in with the code of a healthy cell it is unable to reproduce. In other words, viruses use cells as factories for their own production. Zinc is instrumental in stopping the spread of viruses by preventing their access to the multiplication machinery of the cell.

Zinc's antioxidant properties

Zinc, acting as part of an enzyme with antioxident properties, helps to protect the cells of the immune system from the damaging effects of free radicals. These are highly reactive molecules capable of damaging cellular structures. Free radicals are abundant around fighter cells because they are actually used as ammunition against microbes. In addition, they are formed during the battle between the immune system's fighter cells and the foreign bugs. Hence, free radicals are both necessary and potentially harmful to the immune system.

Zinc's role lies in its ability to help reduce free radical damage to cells of the immune system, while allowing free radical attack against the dangerous microbes. Zinc forms part of an enzyme situated right on the fighter cell's outer membrane; this position makes it possible for the enzyme to disarm the free radicals surrounding the fighter cell which would otherwise come into contact with the cell. Zinc is essential for the enzyme's activity, helping to keep the composition of the cell membrane intact and making the fighter cells stronger.

If your child's diet is low in zinc, in time the zinc present in the cell membranes will become depleted. This will expose the cells to more attacks by free radicals, causing premature and irreversible damage to the cells, ending finally in their destruction and a weakened immunity.

Zinc's role in boosting immunity is supported by many studies. Well designed studies show that zinc supplementation is helpful in reducing the occurrence and duration of infectious diarrhoea in children by up to 30%. Similarly, it has been shown that zinc reduces the occurrence of acute respiratory infections by almost half.

As with most other nutritional supplements zinc supplements will only be of benefit in times of zinc deficiency. Preventing zinc deficiency in children in the first place would be of even greater benefit.

Acute lower respiratory infections

A well designed study published in 1998 in the journal *Pediatrics* looked at the occurrence of acute lower respiratory infections (where the majority of cases were due to pneumonia) in Indian children aged 6–35 months. The study showed that zinc plays a crucial role in determining whether or not children succumb to respiratory infections. The study gave 298 children a supplement of 10 mg of elemental zinc daily for 120 days and compared their progress to a control group of children not given the zinc supplement. The dosage of 10 mg of zinc represents 270%, 200% and 125% of the RDI for children aged 1–3 years, 4–7 years and 8–11 years respectively. After 120 days the children's blood zinc levels were tested, and the number of episodes of acute lower respiratory infections was compared between the two groups.

The results showed that the group of children who were supplemented with zinc had 45% fewer episodes of respiratory infections than before the supplementation. Comparing the two groups of children, it was found that those who were not given the zinc supplement suffered respiratory infections almost twice as often. It is important to note that, after supplementation, only 11.6% of supplemented children, as opposed to 43.6% of unsupplemented children, had low zinc levels shown by blood tests. The study clearly showed that improving zinc intake in infants and school children deficient in zinc significantly reduced the number of respiratory infections they suffered.

Do children consume enough zinc?

A recent report from the United States showed that only 6% of children were consuming the recommended daily amount of zinc, with an alarming 94% of children not getting enough. This is worrying as even mild zinc deficiency has been shown to depress the immune system. A well designed follow-up study which looked at the nutrient and food intake of children over time (from age 24 to 60 months) who were primarily of middle and upper socio-economic status, also found zinc to be lacking in these children's diets. This study compared the zinc intake of the children to the daily recommendations for zinc in the United States, which is set at 10 mg for children—higher than the recommendations in Australia. However, the children in this study did not even meet the Australian RDI set at 6 mg during their third year of life. Since both the United States and the Australian diets are recognised as typically 'Western', the findings of this United States study may also be relevant to Australian children.

The RDI for children in Australia starts at 4.5 mg for children aged 1–3 years, goes up to 6 mg for 4–7 year olds, and increases again to 9 mg for children aged 8–11 years. The most recent National Nutrition Survey, carried out in 1995 on Australian children, did not report low zinc intakes in our children. It is important to note, however, that the survey was based on a one-day food recall. Longer periods of dietary assessment are needed to make a more accurate assessment of children's zinc intakes. Earlier assessments referred to zinc as 'borderline' in the Australian community and, compared with other nutrients, it is relatively hard to supply adequate amounts in a typical mixed diet.

Loss of appetite

Even a mild zinc deficiency may result in impaired taste and smell, and in children this may spoil their enjoyment of food. This can result in fussy eating and lead to a poor food intake overall. This may turn into a vicious circle with lower zinc levels fuelling lower appetites. If you have children who are fussy eaters you may like to review their food choices to make sure their diet is not low in zinc. You will find many quick, tasty recipes at the end of this chapter to help increase the amount of zinc your child is eating.

Food sources of zinc

Good sources of zinc include liver, shellfish, oysters, lean meat, canned fish, hard cheese, whole grains, nuts, eggs and pulses. Vegetables contain smaller amounts of zinc and also contain compounds such as phytates and oxalates, which bind zinc, leaving less available for absorption. The zinc in grains is found mainly in the germ and bran coverings, so food refining and processing reduce the amount of zinc in food. For example, flour refining causes a 77% loss in zinc, rice refining causes a loss of 83% and processing cereals from whole grains causes an 80% loss. The advantage of refined cereals is that they are lower in phytates so more zinc is actually absorbed from refined breads and cereals. In practice, it appears that regardless of whether you offer white or wholegrain bread to children the amount of zinc they will absorb will be roughly the same (but wholegrain breads are high in fibre amongst other nutrients).

The way we prepare foods does, however, make a difference to zinc's availability for absorption. By cooking legumes thoroughly we reduce the ability of phytate's to bind zinc, and so more zinc is absorbed. Bran, which is particularly high in phytates, should not be given to small children. For older children, add some bran to the baking mixture for muffins, fruit breads and fruit cakes. Nuts and wheat germ are two very good sources of zinc and should be used often and in many ways to increase the zinc in a

Table 4.1

Zinc content of foods

Food	Portion	Amount (mg)*
Bread and Cereals		
Bread, white	1 slice	0.2
Oats, cooked	1/2 cup	0.4
Millet	1/2 cup	0.6
Pearl barley	1/2 cup	0.4
Puffed rice cereal	1/2 cup	0.2
Wheat germ	1 tbsp	0.5
Vegetables (cooked)		
Asparagus	1/4 cup	0.1
Beans, Lima, dry	1/4 cup	0.4
Beans, red	1/4 cup	0.5
Broccoli	1/4 cup	0.2
Chickpeas, dry	1/4 cup	0.5
Corn	1/4 cup	0.3
Lentils, dry	1/4 cup	0.4
Okra	1/4 cup	0.3
Peas	1/4 cup	0.3
Seaweed, raw	1/4 cup	0.3
Soybeans, dry	1/4 cup	0.7
Spinach, English	1/4 cup	0.2
Meat and Alternatives (raw)		
Bean curd (tofu)	1/4 cup	0.5
Beef	45 g	1.8
Brazil nuts	1 tbsp	0.5
Cashews, dry roasted	1 tbsp	0.7
Cheese, cheddar	30 g	1.1
Chicken, breast	45 g	0.4
Chicken, thigh	45 g	0.8
Egg	45 g	0.4
Fish	45 g	0.3
Lamb	45 g	1.4
Milk, fluid, whole	1/2 cup	0.5
Peanut butter	1 tbsp	0.7
Pork	45 g	0.9
Pumpkin seeds	1 tbsp	0.7
Sunflower seeds	1 tbsp	0.8
Tahini, sesame butter	1 tbsp	1.0
Veal	45 g	1.3
Yoghurt	100 g	0.5

* RDI for children 1–3 years is 4.5 mg; for children 4–7 years 6 mg; and for children 8–11 years 9 mg.
Source: FoodWorks Professional Edition Copyright 1998–2000 Xyris Software.

child's diet. For small children nuts should be ground to reduce the risk of choking.

The absorption of zinc from dairy foods is more efficient than from plant sources. But the calcium that is present in dairy foods joins hands with phytates and further inhibits the absorption of zinc from plant foods. For this reason, avoid serving dairy products with plant foods that are rich in zinc, such as legumes.

To improve zinc absorption from children's diets:

- Avoid serving cola.
- Avoid serving tea or cocoa with meals.
- Avoid sprinkling raw bran on cereals. Instead, add bran to mixtures for baked products.
- Cook legumes well until very soft.
- Add wheat germ to cereals and into baking mixtures, for example, muffins.

Table 4.1 gives the zinc content of various foods.

Zinc supplements

Zinc supplements given to healthy children did not show any side effects in amounts of twice the daily recommendation, which is set at 10 mg in the United States. Despite these findings, zinc supplementation is not justified in such large doses for children eating a mixed Western diet. Much smaller doses, if any, are more appropriate. We look at zinc supplements in more detail in Chapter 9.

Ingredients

Makes approximately:
12 serves for 1–3 year olds
10 serves for 4–7 year olds
8 serves for 8–11 year olds

250 g cooked shaped pasta

125 g ricotta cheese

3 eggs

1 tablespoon olive oil

1 onion, finely chopped

500 g minced lean chicken

400 g can tomatoes, chopped

½ cup water

2 tablespoons homemade tomato sauce (see recipe on p. 116)

300 ml carton fresh light cream

1½ cups grated cheddar cheese

finely chopped parsley (omit for very young children)

Method

- Preheat oven to 180°C.
- In mixing bowl, mix the pasta, ricotta and 1 egg. Place in a greased baking dish.
- In a frying pan, heat the oil and sauté the onion until soft.
- Add the chicken and cook until it changes colour, stirring frequently.
- Add the tomatoes, water and tomato sauce.
- Simmer until sauce thickens, about 20 minutes, and then pour over the pasta mixture.
- Beat the remaining eggs with the cream.
- Mix in the cheese and spoon over the chicken mixture.
- Sprinkle with parsley.
- Bake for 30 minutes.

Nutritional analysis per serve

Zinc
Age 1–3 years: 1.70 mg—40% RDI
Age 4–7 years: 2.10 mg—34% RDI
Age 8–11 years: 2.57 mg—28% RDI

Baking increases zinc absorption from flours and grains.

Ingredients

Makes 12 muffins

1 1/2 cups whole-wheat flour

1 cup unbleached all-purpose flour

1/2 cup sugar

1 teaspoon bicarbonate of soda

1 teaspoon baking powder

1/2 teaspoon salt

1/4 teaspoon ground allspice

1 cup buttermilk

2 tablespoons olive oil

1 large egg white

1 3/4 cups fresh or thawed frozen blueberries

Method

- Preheat oven to 190°C.
- Line 12 standard-size muffin pan cups with foil muffin cups.
- In a small bowl, combine whole-wheat flour, all-purpose flour, sugar, baking soda, baking powder, salt and allspice.
- In a medium bowl, whisk together buttermilk, oil and egg white.
- Add dry ingredients to buttermilk mixture, stirring until just moistened.
- Gently fold in blueberries.
- Spoon batter into muffin cups, filling each about two-thirds full.
- Bake for 20–25 minutes or until tops are lightly golden.
- Set pan on a wire rack for 5 minutes.
- Turn muffins out onto rack and cool completely.

Nutritional analysis per serve

Zinc
Age 1–3 years: 0.4 mg—8% RDI
Age 4–7 years: 0.4 mg—7% RDI
Age 8–11 years: 0.4 mg—4% RDI

Ingredients

Makes approximately:
8 serves for 1–3 year olds
6 serves for 4–7 year olds
4 serves for 8–11 year olds

1 tablespoon olive oil

120 g onions, diced

450 g beef, thinly sliced

120 g broccoli, chopped

120 g cauliflower, chopped

120 g green beans, sliced

Method

- Sauté onions in olive oil until slightly brown, then add meat.
- When meat is almost cooked, add a small amount of water and the vegetables.
- Cover and cook for 1 minute.
- Remove cover and continue cooking for 5 more minutes.
- Do not overcook the vegetables.

Nutritional analysis per serve

Zinc
Age 1–3 years: 2.4 mg—50% RDI
Age 4–7 years: 3.2 mg—50% RDI
Age 8–11 years: 4.8 mg—50% RDI

Ingredients

Makes approximately:
8 serves for 1–3 year olds
6 serves for 4–7 year olds
4 serves for 8–11 year olds

1 x 425 g can tuna

1 cup cooked peas

2 hard-boiled eggs

1 cup white sauce (see below) with 2 tablespoons of grated cheddar cheese mixed in

500 g potatoes, cooked and mashed

1 cup grated cheddar cheese

White sauce

1 tablespoon monounsaturated margarine

3 teaspoons white flour

1 cup milk

Method

- To make sauce, melt margarine then add flour, mixing well to a smooth paste to make a roux. Cool. Bring milk to the boil then allow to cool for a few minutes. Gradually pour milk into the roux, mixing well with a wooden spoon to avoid lumps. If lumps form, pass through a fine strainer.
- Drain tuna, flake with fork and place in a buttered casserole dish.
- Add peas, halved hard-boiled eggs and white sauce mixture.
- Cover with mashed potato and top with grated cheese.
- Bake in a moderate oven for 20 minutes.

Nutritional analysis per serve

Zinc
Age 1–3 years: 1.7 mg—35% RDI
Age 4–7 years: 2.2 mg—35% RDI
Age 8–11 years: 3.3 mg—35% RDI

Ingredients

Makes approximately:
8 serves for 1–3 year olds
6 serves for 4–7 year olds
4 serves for 8–11 year olds

2 teaspoons olive oil

1 carrot, sliced

1 small parsnip, sliced

1 stick celery, sliced

1 cup water

500 g lean pork fillets

2 tablespoons cornflour

1–3 tablespoons plum sauce

Method

- In a medium saucepan heat oil for 1 minute over a high heat.
- Add vegetables and stir-fry for 3–5 minutes.
- Add meat and stir-fry for 5 minutes.
- Blend cornflour with a little water to form a smooth paste.
- Add to casserole, and stir well.
- Cook over a medium heat for 2 minutes.
- Stir in plum sauce to taste.
- Garnish with 2 stalks of spring onions, diagonally chopped, and serve with rice.

Nutritional analysis per serve

Zinc
Age 1–3 years: 1.2 mg—25% RDI
Age 4–7 years: 1.5 mg—25% RDI
Age 8–11 years: 2.3 mg—25% RDI

Ingredients

Makes 10 burgers

500 g premium minced beef

200 g carrot, grated

200 g zucchini, grated

200 g granny smith apples, grated

400 g potatoes, peeled, grated

1 cup breadcrumbs firmly packed

2 tablespoons wholemeal plain flour

1/4 cup fresh parsley, finely chopped

1/2 teaspoon nutmeg

1/2 teaspoon dried mixed herbs

Method

- Combine all ingredients and mix with hands.
- Shape into equal size balls.
- Flatten balls, and place in a lightly greased pan and cook on moderate heat for approximately 6 minutes.
- Carefully turn over and cook for a further 4–5 minutes.
- Remove from pan and place on absorbent paper for a few minutes.
- Divide a wholemeal burger bun or use 2 wholemeal pita breads.
- Add shredded lettuce, onion rings, tomato slices, grated carrot, red and green capsicum rings, bean sprouts.
- Top with tomato chutney or tomato sauce.

Nutritional analysis per serve

Zinc
Age 1–3 years: 3 mg—65% RDI
Age 4–7 years: 3 mg—50% RDI
Age 8–11 years: 3 mg—33% RDI

Substitute smooth peanut butter for crunchy for children under 5 years of age.

Ingredients

Makes approximately:
4 serves for 1–3 year olds
3 serves for 4–7 year olds
2 serves for 8–11 year olds

250 g chicken fillets, chopped
2 teaspoons olive oil
1 small onion, chopped
1 clove garlic
1½ tablespoons crunchy peanut butter
¼ cup chicken stock
1½ tablespoons soy sauce
1½ tablespoons water
1 tablespoon honey
½ teaspoon curry powder
¼ teaspoon ginger powder

Method

- Heat oil.
- Cook onion, garlic and ginger until onion is soft.
- Mix together remaining ingredients (except chicken) and add to onion mixture.
- Place chicken in casserole dish and pour mixture over chicken pieces.
- Cook at 180°C for approximately 1 hour, cover with foil after ½ hour.

Nutritional analysis per serve

Zinc
Age 1–3 years: 1.6 mg—35% RDI
Age 4–7 years: 2.1 mg—35% RDI
Age 8–11 years: 3.1 mg—35% RDI

Ingredients

500 g finely minced veal

1 onion, grated

1 tablespoon oyster sauce

1 tablespoon soy sauce

1 egg, beaten

olive oil for cooking

Makes approximately:
8 serves for 1–3 year olds
6 serves for 4–7 year olds
4 serves for 8–11 year olds

Method

- Combine all the ingredients in a bowl.
- Roll into balls with clean, cold hands.
- Cook in frying pan in a little heated oil over a medium heat, turning until brown and cooked through.
- Drain on kitchen paper before serving.

Nutritional analysis per serve

Zinc
Age 1–3 years: 1.9 mg—45% RDI
Age 4–7 years: 2.6 mg—45% RDI
Age 8–11 years: 3.9 mg—45% RDI

Attractive to look at and guaranteed to be eaten.

Ingredients

Makes approximately:
6 serves for 1–3 year olds
4 serves for 4–7 year olds
3 serves for 8–11 year olds

175 g light cream cheese or ricotta cheese

2 tablespoons chives, chopped

1/4 cup parsley leaves

3 teaspoons mustard, mild

3 pieces lavash bread

225 g lean leg ham

Method

- Blend cheese, chives, parsley and mustard in a food processor until smooth.
- Spread the lavash bread evenly with the mixture.
- Place ham onto the spread.
- Roll bread over the filling tightly.
- Wrap around to form a firm roll.
- To serve, cut the lavash into 1½ cm thick diagonal slices.

Nutritional analysis per serve

Zinc
Age 1–3 years: 1.2 mg—25% RDI
Age 4–7 years: 1.8 mg—30% RDI
Age 8–11 years: 2.4 mg—25% RDI

Ingredients

Makes approximately:
4 serves for 1–3 year olds
3 serves for 4–7 year olds
2 serves for 8–11 year olds

120 g chicken mince, raw

200 ml chicken stock

1/2 teaspoon minced fresh ginger root
or 1/4 teaspoon ginger powder

125 g or one small can creamed sweet corn

1 small egg, well beaten

1–2 teaspoons cornflour, mixed well with water

Method

- Stir chicken mince into cold stock and add ginger and sweet corn.
- Bring to boil and simmer for 30 minutes.
- Add cornflour while stirring and boil for 2 minutes.
- While boiling, rapidly stir in beaten eggs and whisk with a fork.
- Serve at once.

Nutritional analysis per serve

Zinc
Age 1–3 years: 0.5 mg—10 % RDI
Age 4–7 years: 0.6 mg—10 % RDI
Age 8–11 years: 0.9 mg—10 % RDI

5
Antioxidants versus free radicals

Free radicals are extremely reactive molecules that attract healthy molecules through small electric charges, rather like a static comb attracts hair. Free radicals exert many damaging effects on the cells of the immune system because they actually change the chemistry of molecules. One major concern is their damaging effect on the cell membranes of the fighter cells. Damage to the membranes renders the cells less able to combat infections. Free radicals can also damage the DNA blueprint of the fighter cells. The DNA blueprint can be likened to a recipe for a dish. It holds the instructions on how to make the fighter cells from its constituents, just like making a dish from its many ingredients. Damage to the DNA of the fighter cells may result in inferior fighter cells just as omitting one ingredient may result in a less tasty dish.

The good news is that there are nutrients in certain foods that limit or prevent the damage done by free radicals. A well balanced diet can be a rich source of nutrients that are capable of stopping these harmful reactions from taking place. These nutrients are called *antioxidants.*

Three nutrients in particular are crucial in the fight against free radicals: vitamins C and E, and beta carotene. Trace metals selenium, copper and zinc are also important in the fight against free radicals, as they form part of enzymes with antioxidant properties. Finally, plant chemicals called *flavonoids* show strong antioxidant properties.

Studies show that antioxidant levels fall during infections. Scientists think that they are being used up fighting free radicals. There seems to be a race going on between free radicals and antioxidants. The free radicals are generated at a faster rate during infection and the antioxidants are trying to keep up and prevent their damaging effects. Which group will come out on top depends on the blood levels of antioxidants and this in turn depends on how much antioxidants children consume.

Prevention of viral infections

Scientists have known for some time that a deficiency in the nutrients that are important to a healthy immune system brings about a slower and less effective immune response. At such times infections are more likely to occur and are more severe. New evidence shows that it is not only the immune system that undergoes changes during times of poor nutrition. Researchers studying the behaviour of viruses found that a deficiency of antioxidant nutrients resulted in mutations or changes at the genetic level of the virus. These changes produce a more virulent and more infective virus. These mutations can be likened to a switching mechanism whereby the virus is switched on to a highly infective type.

Although the studies did not focus on the cold sore virus, this virus seems to demonstrate this new evidence. The cold sore virus is normally dormant and there are no physical signs of its presence. It flares up, however, from time to time, erupting in a painful mouth sore. It is then highly contagious. Flare-up usually occur when the immune system is 'down'. Providing a diet rich in antioxidants will prevent the free radical formation that stresses the immune system and allows viruses to take a foothold. One indication of antioxidant involvement is the fall in antioxidant levels during infections when they are being used up fighting free radicals.

Let's look at each antioxidant nutrient in more detail.

Vitamin C

Vitamin C is a powerful free radical quencher; it protects the fighter cells involved in the battle against colds, flu and other infections. It offers protection by quenching the highly reactive chemicals before they damage the physical structure of the fighter cells. In addition to its role as a powerful antioxidant, vitamin C is essential for the body's production of antibodies, and for the healthy function of white blood cells. It plays an important role in the production of interferon, the chemical messenger that prevents viruses from gaining a foothold, and is also involved in the detection and destruction of cancerous cells.

The common cold

Vitamin C has long been thought to prevent and even help cure the common cold. The evidence is not conclusive, although many studies support the role of vitamin C in shortening the duration of cold symptoms, particularly a blocked and runny nose. Vitamin C reduces the histamines that circulate in the blood, triggering tissue inflammation and a runny nose.

Vitamin C's most prominent advocate was Dr Linus Pauling who believed that vitamin C in large 1-gram doses reduced the incidence of the common cold by 45%. Since then, many studies have looked at the role of vitamin C in combating the common cold. Some well designed and some less well designed studies came up with sometimes contradictory findings. Recently, they were critically reviewed, and the following conclusions were reached:

- *The incidence of the common cold.* Increasing the amount of Vitamin C in your child's diet will reduce the number of times your child suffers from a common cold *only* if your child's diet is low in vitamin C.

- *The duration and severity of the common cold.* A study in Sweden on 615 school children showed that children who received a regular vitamin C supplement missed significantly fewer school days than children without vitamin C supplementation. Overall, studies in Europe show that vitamin C supplementation during winter, when consumption of fresh fruit rich in vitamin C is likely to be poor, helps to reduce the severity and duration of the common cold in children and adults, most likely due to the correction of marginal deficiencies.

- *Other respiratory infections.* Vitamin C proved helpful in the fight against streptococci bacteria, which cause tonsillitis infections in children. When schoolboys with a marginal deficiency of vitamin C were given a supplement of between 50 and 600 milligrams of vitamin C daily (which represents a range from just over one RDI to eleven times the daily recommended amount of vitamin C), they required less hospitalisation and recovered more quickly from tonsillitis. The schoolboys in this study were eating on average 15 milligrams of vitamin C daily, which is half the recommended daily dose for children, and clearly not enough. Data on vitamin C intakes in Australian children has found significantly better results, with the most recent National Nutrition Survey (1995) finding adequate vitamin C consumption.

A study looking at the incidence of wheeze and chronic bronchitis in children found that children with higher blood levels of vitamin C on average suffered fewer episodes of bronchitis and less wheeze.

Sources of vitamin C

Making sure your child consumes enough vitamin C is fairly easy—start with citrus fruit or any fruit rich in vitamin C. Browse through Table 5.1 for other food sources rich in this vitamin.

Table 5.1

Vitamin C content of foods

Food	Portion	Amount (mg)*
Fruits (raw)		
Grapefruit	1/2 small	25
Guava	1/2 medium	108
Kiwifruit	1 medium	57
Lychee	6 medium	30
Mango	1/2 medium	28
Orange	1 small	50
Pawpaw	1/2 cup	45
Pineapple	1/2 cup	17
Strawberry	1/4 cup	18
Vegetables (cooked)		
Broccoli	1/4 cup	43
Brussels sprouts	1/4 cup	36
Vegetables (raw)		
Capsicum	1/4 cup	33
Tomato	1/2 small	10
Tomato, cherry	3 medium	14

* RDI for all children: 30 mg

Source: FoodWorks Professional Edition, Copyright 1988–2000 Xyris Software.

Vitamin E

Vitamin E is invaluable as a scavenger of free radicals in cell membranes. It prevents the destruction of membranes of the many globules which contain toxic free radicals and are used like bullets against microbes, which are present inside the fighter cells. In addition to its role as an antioxidant, vitamin E offers protection to the thymus gland, a vital organ where the manufacture of white cells takes place. It also protects fighter cells as they do their job.

Vitamin E is fat-loving and snuggles into lipid or fat environments around the body. It is found in the membranes of cells which are a mixture of different molecules submerged in a layer of fatty acids. Vitamin E is essential to keep the structure of the lipid membranes intact, which in turn protect the internal contents of the cells. Vitamin E is particularly important for membrane protection of the immune cells for their membranes contain unusually high amounts of polyunsaturated fatty acids which are particularly susceptible to damage by the free radicals. Damage to fighter cell membranes renders the cells less efficient at accomplishing their tasks within the tight network of reactions to prevent infection.

Vitamin E has been shown to be particularly important in times of illness when oxidative stress occurs—for example, during chronic viral infections. Studies are now under way to look at the amounts of vitamin E that may be needed to compensate for the body's higher needs for vitamin E during infections. Some results are already available. In one study of adults scientists found that supplementing with 268 milligrams of vitamin E for three days helped phagocytic cells like macrophages (cells that gobble up germs) do so more quickly, and this prevented the spread of the bacteria. This and other preliminary studies have researchers thinking that it may be beneficial to recommend a higher amount of vitamin E during times of infection. The supplemented dose of vitamin E in this and other studies represents a large amount in comparison to the daily recommendation for children, roughly 30 times higher. It is impractical to obtain this amount of vitamin E from the diet without supplementation.

Because the studies are preliminary and to date have involved only adults we must be cautious when applying the findings to children. Researchers are very excited, however, and are devising studies to show just how much vitamin E is optimal for the immune system. Let's hope they search for the optimal immune-boosting amount for children as well. For now I do not recommend supplementing children with large doses of vitamin E. However, a more moderate supplemental dose around the RDI for children may be helpful for children who suffer from frequent infections.

We now look at how much dietary vitamin E is recommended for children daily and how to incorporate it into daily food choices.

Food sources of vitamin E

The best sources of vitamin E are wheat germ, seeds and nuts, particularly almonds, and avocado and soybeans. Table 5.2 lists the good sources of vitamin E.

When looking at the content of vitamin E in foods we need to consider how much polyunsaturated fat they contain. Eating polyunsaturated fats increases children's need for vitamin E: the more polyunsaturated fats they consume the more vitamin E they need. Vitamin E is vital to help the fats remain stable and keep their natural structure. Hence, eating a food that is rich in both vitamin E and polyunsaturated fats means that the vitamin E will be used up to maintain the structure of the dietary fats, and not much can be spared to guard the immune system against free radicals. So, when choosing oils (which are rich in fats), we should select those that have a good ratio of vitamin E to polyunsaturated fats. Two oils fit this description—olive oil and sunflower oil—these oils contain the best ratio of vitamin E to polyunsaturated oils.

Table 5.2

Vitamin E content of foods

Food	Amount (mg ATE)*
Wheat germ, 2 tbsp	3.4
Vegetables (1/2 cup cooked unless otherwise indicated)	
Asparagus	0.3
Avocado, 1/2 raw	1.3
Cabbage	0.1
Parsnips	0.4
Pumpkin	1.3
Stewed tomatoes	0.7
Sweet potato	0.5
Fruits (raw)	
Mango	0.9
Pear	0.4
Legumes	
Soybeans, 1/2 cup cooked	1.6
Nuts/seeds (30 g)	
Almonds	7.4
Brazil nuts	2.2
Peanuts	3.2
Peanut butter	3.2
Sunflower seeds	15.0
Walnuts	0.8
Vegetable oils (1 tbsp)	
Margarine, 1 tsp	2.4
Mayonnaise	0.6
Olive oil	1.7
Sunflower oil	6.8

* Alpha Tocopherols Equivalents. RDI of vitamin E for 1–3 year olds is 5 mg ATE; for 4–7 year olds 6 mg ATE; and for 8–11 year olds 8 mg ATE.

Selenium

Selenium forms part of glutathione peroxidase, an enzyme with strong antioxidant properties. The role of glutathione peroxidase is the protection of white blood cells, and their speedy production should the need for more arise. This selenium dependant enzyme is also known to enhance the action of the fighter cells.

Selenium helps vitamin E in the fight against free radicals. Vitamin E and selenium work in different ways to reduce or prevent the damage caused by free radicals. Despite their different action, they cooperate by sparing one another, both working as antioxidants. If selenium is low in your child's diet vitamin E will step in and take over some of its work. In the same way, selenium can spare some of the vitamin E. It is best, however, to look after the

Table 5.3

Selenium content of foods

Food	Amount (mcg)*
Bread, cereals, grains	
Bread, white, 1 slice	6
Bread, whole-wheat, 1 slice	8
English muffin, 1/2	14
Oatmeal, 1/2 cup cooked	10
Pearl barley, 1/2 cup cooked	7
Rice, white, 1/2 cup cooked	6
Legumes	
Lentils, cooked 1/2 cup	3
Nuts/seeds	
Brazil nuts, 30 g	840
Animal products	
Egg, 1 large	18

* RDI for children 1–3 years is 25 mcg; for 4-7 years 30 mcg; for 8-11 years 50 mcg.
Source: USDA Nutrient Database for Standard Reference.

child's nutritional need for both selenium and vitamin E to optimise the antioxidant action of both. Table 5.3 lists selenium values of common foods.

Copper

Copper itself has no known antioxidant properties but it forms part of a powerful complex molecule that plays a crucial role in neutralising free radicals. This powerful molecule is the enzyme, copper superoxide dismutase, the hard worker against free radical damage. There are many types of superoxide dismutase, as you may have realised by now. Some require zinc, some need selenium and some depend on copper. Copper stands out among the other metals because the latest research links it with the genetic machinery responsible for the production of all superoxide dismutases. It appears that copper is crucial for the right molecular machinery to attach itself to the genetic code and start the process by which these enzymes are actually made.

Copper also plays a vital part in the activation of T cells. Diets low in copper, which cause low copper blood levels, are responsible for the less efficient functioning of these fighter cells.

To date there is no recommended daily amount for copper in children's diets so it is difficult to comment on their consumption of copper. Good sources of copper include brazil nuts, tahini, sunflower seeds, peanut butter, avocado and soybeans.

Flavonoids and children's immunity

Fruits, vegetables, cocoa and tea in some cultures are the major sources of flavonoids in children's diets. Flavonoids are found in the edible pulp of fruits such as citrus fruits, apricots, cherries, grapes, blackcurrants, berries and rosehips. In the vegetable kingdom green pepper (capsicum), broccoli, onions and tomatoes are good sources, and buckwheat is also a rich source. Green tea is an excellent source of several flavonoids; black tea is less rich but also a good source. Earlier, there were doubts about whether flavonoids can be absorbed into the body but it is now accepted that flavonoids are usually easily absorbed and play a major role in preventing free radical damage.

Flavonoids are able to guard the immune system due to their unique chemistry. They are able to disarm free radicals and reactive chemical entities that would otherwise chemically change and damage structural components in the body. They help to guard the cellular components of the immune system during oxidative stress, a time when more free radicals are generated—for example, during respiratory infections.

Flavonoids also work in partnership with other antioxidants. Flavonoids help the antioxidant vitamins, C and E, to do their work. They have a synergistic action, which means that together they can achieve more to help boost the immune system. Flavonoids, and particularly citrus flavonoids, are often given with vitamin C supplements, for example in the treatment of colds. In nature, citrus fruits are a great source of both vitamin C and flavonoids.

Fresh fruit helps breathing

A study in England, which surveyed 2650 children, revealed that eating fresh fruit helps children to breathe more easily. The researchers measured the children's forced expiratory volume in one second by getting the children to breathe out as hard as they could into a device that measured the volume of the air they expired. By relating the measurements to the amount of fresh fruit the children ate on a daily basis, the researchers found that:

- children who ate more fresh fruit were able to breathe out more air, and
- this was seen more often in children who suffered from wheezing.

They concluded that:

- eating fresh fruit helps lung function in children.

The study also found that eating vegetables and fresh vegetable salads had a similarly helpful effect. Now what's so special about fruit and vegetables? They are full of flavonoids as well as vitamin C. The Australian National Nutrition Survey in 1995 showed that approximately one-third of children aged 3–11 years had not eaten any fruit on the day of the survey. Furthermore, one in five children had not eaten fresh vegetables or any vegetable products that day.

Antioxidant levels in the diet

Should we be concerned about the levels of antioxidants in children's diets?

Children get sufficient vitamin C in a typical Western diet but the source of it is less than ideal. Studies have shown that children get most of their vitamin C from fruit juices that are fortified with vitamin C.

Some studies from the United States report poor intakes of vitamin E in young children. The National Nutrition Survey (1995) did not look at the vitamin E intakes of the Australian population and hence it shows no vitamin E intakes for Australian children.

Selenium intake depends largely on the soil content of the regions where food crops are grown, and the selenium content of vegetables and grains may vary greatly across the continent. It is difficult to make good estimations for the selenium content of children's diets, and I am not aware of any relevant nutritional studies in Australian children.

Preliminary reports from the United States say that the typical Western diet (which would include the Australian diet) contains less copper than the amounts set as the Estimated Safe and Adequate Daily Dietary Intake (ESADDI) for all age groups including children. Set in the United States, the ESADDI are only provisional recommended allowances as more research is needed to validate the recommendations. There is no copper RDI set for children in Australia and, as a result, copper is not included in the regular national nutrition surveys. Hence, it is impossible to evaluate whether Australian children are getting sufficient copper in their diet.

There is very limited data on the intake of flavonoids, and none that I am aware of in children. However, both the National Nutrition Survey and reports from overseas clearly show that children are not eating enough fruits and vegetables in their diets. And as children grow older they tend to eat less fruit. As fruit and vegetables are the best sources of flavonoids this points to a low supply of flavonoids in children's diets.

Chocolate was heralded as an excellent source of antioxidants in 2000. Chocolate owes its high antioxidant content to the cocoa plant, which is a major ingredient in chocolate. Cocoa liquor is rich in polyphenols, including quercetin and epicatechin. *Polyphenols* inhibit two major classes of free radicals, hydrogen peroxide and superoxides. There is no advantage to eating chocolate over drinking cocoa powder in the form of hot chocolate. Cocoa powder contains 20 mg of total phenol gallic acid per gram, cooking chocolate contains 8.4 mg per gram and milk chocolate contains 5 mg per gram. A cup of hot chocolate made with approximately two tablespoons of cocoa powder contains 146 mg of phenols, while a 40 gram chocolate bar contains approximately 205 mg.

Chocolate contains a lot more kilojoules because of its high fat and sugar content. Therefore, despite its high antioxidant content, it is not a food to offer as a means of providing your children with antioxidants. Chocolate should remain a treat food. Cocoa powder, on the other hand, can be added at home in many nutritious ways to both foods and drinks. Note that artificial chocolate flavouring does not contain cocoa and has no beneficial antioxidant properties.

The recipe section includes tempting ways to ensure a steady supply of fruit and vegetables in your child's diet. Table 5.4 lists the best sources of antioxidants.

Table 5.4

Top antioxidant fruits and vegetables

Food item	**ORAC***
Prunes	5770
Raisins	2830
Blueberries	2400
Blackberries	2036
Strawberries	1540
Spinach	1260
Raspberries	1220
Brussels sprouts	980
Plums	949
Alfalfa sprouts	930
Broccoli florets	890
Oranges	750
Grapes, red	739
Capsicum, red	710
Cherries	670
Onion	450
Corn	400
Eggplant	390

* ORAC—Oxygen Radical Absorbance Capacity—a measure of the ability of foods to subdue harmful oxygen-free radicals. ORAC units per 100g.

Source: US Department of Agriculture.

Grind cashew nuts for children younger than 5 years of age. The seasoning is mild and adds to the flavour of the dish.

Ingredients

Makes approximately 10 serves

1 teaspoon olive oil
1 large carrot, thinly sliced
100 g cauliflower, broken into very small florets
175 g cabbage, chopped into 2.5 cm lengths
pinch of chilli powder
pinch of ginger powder
1 teaspoon honey
2 teaspoons soy sauce
150 ml vegetable stock
2 teaspoons wine vinegar
1 teaspoon sesame seeds, crushed
1 teaspoon cornflour
100 g bean shoots, rinsed well under tap
50 g cashew nuts, whole or in pieces, toasted under a low grill for a few minutes

Method

- Heat the oil in a large frying pan or wok.
- Add the carrot and stir-fry for 2–3 minutes.
- Add the cauliflower and cook for another 2–3 minutes.
- Add chilli and ginger powders.
- Combine the honey, soy sauce, stock, vinegar, sesame seeds, and cornflour.
- Pour this mixture over the vegetables, cover the pan and simmer for 3 minutes.
- Add the bean shoots and cook for 1 minute.
- Serve with cashew nuts sprinkled on top.

Nutritional analysis per serve

Selenium
Age 1–3 years: 14 mcg—55% RDI
Age 4–7 years: 14 mcg—50% RDI
Age 8–11 years: 14 mcg—30% RDI

Copper
1.6 mg

Vitamin E
Age 1–3 years: 2 mg ATE—40% RDI
Age 4–7 years: 2 mg ATE—30% RDI
Age 8–11 years: 2 mg ATE—25% RDI

A great combination of vegetables and the immunity-boosting nutrients vitamin E, selenium and copper.

Ingredients

Makes approximately 5 serves

1 cup macaroni

1 cup diced carrot

1 cup green beans cut into 2 cm lengths

1 cup green peas

2 zucchini, diced

2 tablespoons butter

2 tablespoons flour

2 cups milk

chopped parsley

1/4–1/2 cup wholemeal breadcrumbs

1 cup grated cheddar cheese

Method

- Cook macaroni according to the instructions on the packet. Drain.
- Steam or microwave vegetables until just tender.
- Make sauce by melting the butter in a pan, add flour and cook, stirring for 2 minutes.
- Add milk gradually, stirring constantly.
- Stir in chopped parsley.
- Layer macaroni, vegetables and sauce in a casserole dish.
- Sprinkle over crumbs and cheese.
- Bake for 30 minutes at 180°C.

Nutritional analysis per serve	*Selenium*	*Vitamin E*
	Age 1–3 years: 45 mcg—180% RDI	Age 1–3 years: 0.5 mg ATE—10% RDI
	Age 4–7 years: 45 mcg—150% RDI	Age 4–7 years: 0.5 mcg ATE— 8% RDI
	Age 8–11 years: 45 mcg— 95% RDI	Age 8–11 years: 0.5 mcg ATE— 6% RDI
	Copper	
	0.6 mg	

Prunes top the list of fruits rich in antioxidants. They are excellent with custard, creamed rice or yoghurt, and because they are soft they are suitable for young children as well. You may blend them if you like and pour to make swirls in custard or yoghurt.

Ingredients

Makes approximately 1–2 serves

4 prunes

1/2 cup water

Method

- Pit prunes.
- Put prunes in a small saucepan.
- Add enough water to cover and simmer over low heat for about 10 minutes.
- The prunes should be tender but still hold their shape.

Nutritional analysis per serve	*Vitamin E*
	Age 1–3 years: 0.5 mg ATE—10% RDI (5% if 2 serves)
	Age 4–7 years: 0.5 mg ATE— 8% RDI
	Age 8–11 years: 0.5 mg ATE— 6% RDI

Much more nutritious than commercial jelly and has a great fresh taste.

Ingredients

Makes approximately 4 serves

4 teaspoons gelatine

3 tablespoons hot water

$1\frac{1}{2}$ teaspoons honey

450 ml orange juice, unsweetened

Method

- Dissolve the gelatine in the hot water with the honey, stirring until it is completely clear.
- Add the gelatine mixture to the juice and stir it in well.
- Chill to set.

Nutritional analysis per serve

Vitamin C
For children of all ages: 40 mg—135% RDI

Ingredients

Makes approximately 8 serves

750 g tomatoes

1 clove garlic

2 tablespoons finely chopped fresh parsley

3 tablespoons olive oil

3 cups chicken stock

2 tablespoons tomato paste

1 cup grated zucchini (optional)

Method

- Chop tomatoes and place in a saucepan with garlic, herbs and olive oil.
- Cook gently for about 5 minutes.
- Add stock and tomato paste and cook for a further 5 minutes.
- If you are using grated zucchini, add 2 minutes before the end of cooking time—no sooner or the zucchini will lose its crunch.

Nutritional analysis per serve

Vitamin C
For children of all ages: 22 mg—70% RDI

Ingredients

Makes approximately 4 serves

2 medium-large ripe tomatoes, peeled and chopped

1 level tablespoon ground rice

1 teaspoon finely chopped chives

pinch of basil powder

pinch of oregano powder

1/4 cup chicken stock

Method

- Put tomatoes and ground rice in a medium saucepan.
- Stir to mix, then add fresh chives and dried herbs.
- Stir, cook over a medium heat for 3–4 minutes to blend seasonings.
- Stir in chicken stock, cover and simmer over a low heat until mixture thickens, approximately 5–6 minutes, stirring twice.
- Sieve, then cool and chill until required.

Nutritional analysis per serve

Vitamin C
For children of all ages: 18 mg—60% RDI

You can replace raspberries with any berries of your choice. All berries are great sources of antioxidants and make yummy fruit smoothies. Frozen, unsweetened berries are readily available in supermarkets. To make a banana smoothie, replace berries with two medium, ripe bananas.

Ingredients

Makes approximately:
5 serves for 1–3 year olds
3 serves for older children

300 g frozen raspberries, thawed

300 ml milk

2 tablespoons sugar

1 teaspoon vanilla extract

1/2 cup ice-cream

Method

- Blend all ingredients together well.

Nutritional analysis per serve
Vitamin C
Age 1–3 years: 12 mg—40% RDI
Older children: 20 mg—65% RDI

Ingredients

Makes approximately:
8 serves for 1–3 year olds
6 serves for 4–7 year olds
4 serves for 8–11 year olds

500 g pork mince

1 egg, beaten

1 cup fresh breadcrumbs

1 carrot, grated

1 apple, peeled and grated

1 tablespoon chopped chives

Method

- Preheat oven to 190°C.
- Mix pork, eggs, breadcrumbs and carrot together thoroughly.
- Add apple and chives to meat and mix well.
- Press into a loaf pan and cook at 190°C for 30–35 minutes.
- Stand to cool for 5 minutes before inverting onto serving plate and slicing.

Nutritional analysis per serve	*Vitamin E*	*Selenium*
	Age 1–3 years: 0.4 mg ATE— 8% RDI	Age 1–3 years: 2.5 mcg—10% RD
	Age 4–7 years: 0.5 mg ATE— 8% RDI	Age 4–7 years: 3.3 mcg—11% RD
	Age 8–11 years: 0.8 mg ATE—10% RDI	Age 8–11 years: 5.0 mcg—10% RD

Ingredients

Makes approximately 5 serves

2 carrots, cut into 1 cm rounds

1 cup cauliflower florets

2 potatoes, peeled and cubed

1/2 cup green beans

3/4 cup water

1 teaspoon fresh lemon juice

3 tablespoons grated unsweetened coconut

1–2 teaspoons curry powder

1/2 cup plain yoghurt, at room temperature

salt to taste

1 3/4 cups water

1 cup uncooked basmati rice

Method

- In a medium saucepan, combine the carrots, cauliflower, potatoes, green beans and 3/4 cup water.
- Cover and cook over medium heat until the vegetables are tender but not mushy, about 15 minutes.
- Add the lemon juice, coconut and curry powder and gradually stir the yoghurt into the vegetable mixture.
- Season with salt.
- In another saucepan, bring the 1 3/4 cups water to a boil.
- Add the rice, cover and simmer until the liquid is absorbed, about 15 minutes.
- Serve the curry over the rice.

Nutritional analysis per serve

Vitamin C
For children of all ages: 30 mg—100% RDI

Selenium
For children of all ages: 10 mcg—approx. 20% RDI

Ingredients

Makes approximately:
8 serves for 1–3 year olds
6 serves for 4–7 year olds
4 serves for 8–11 year olds

2 potatoes

2 or 3 carrots

500 g pumpkin

1 cup green beans

1 choko

1 dessertspoon margarine or butter

1 dessertspoon wholemeal flour

2 cups milk

1 cup grated cheese

½ cup wheat germ

Method

- Steam all vegetables till tender, place in layers in greased casserole dish.
- Melt margarine or butter in saucepan, remove from heat and stir in flour, cook gently for 1 minute.
- Gradually stir in milk and grated cheese until sauce thickens.
- Pour cheese sauce over vegetables and cover top with wheat germ.
- Dot with margarine or butter and bake uncovered until wheat germ is brown.

Nutritional analysis per serve	*Vitamin E*	*Selenium*
	Age 1–3 years: 2.2 mg ATE—45% RDI	Age 1–3 years: 16 mcg
	Age 4–7 years: 2.8 mg ATE—47% RDI	Age 4–7 years: 21 mcg
	Age 8–11 years: 4.3 mg ATE—54% RDI	Age 8–11 years: 32 mcg

Ingredients

Makes approximately:
8 serves for 1–3 year olds
6 serves for 4–7 year olds
4 serves for 8–11 year olds

1 x 440 g can kidney beans, rinsed

1 x 440 g can chickpeas, rinsed

1 medium onion, cut in half and sliced thinly

1 clove garlic, minced

1 teaspoon dried oregano, crumbled

1 teaspoon chilli powder

dash of salt and freshly ground black pepper

1/4 teaspoon cayenne pepper or to taste

2 medium carrots, thinly sliced on the diagonal

1 green or red capsicum, cored and chopped

1/2 cup whole-kernel corn or other vegetable of your choice

1 x 880 g can diced tomatoes

1 cup uncooked couscous

Method

- Combine all the ingredients except the couscous in a medium pot and cook over medium heat until vegetables soften, about 30 minutes.
- Stir in the couscous, cover and remove from the heat.
- Allow to sit 5–10 minutes before serving.

Nutritional analysis per serve

Vitamin E
Age 1–3 years: 0.8 mg ATE—16% RDI
Age 4–7 years: 1.1 mg ATE—18% RDI
Age 8–11 years: 1.4 mg ATE—18% RDI

Ingredients

Makes approximately 8 serves

$^{1}/_{2}$ medium onion, chopped
1 clove garlic, chopped
2 teaspoons shallots, chopped
1 large stalk celery, chopped
1 carrot, diced
$^{1}/_{2}$ cup shredded Savoy cabbage
1 large zucchini, chopped
2$^{1}/_{2}$ cups chicken stock
4 medium tomatoes
1$^{1}/_{2}$ tablespoons tomato paste
1 tablespoon chopped fresh parsley
$^{1}/_{2}$ teaspoon thyme, dried
$^{1}/_{2}$ teaspoon oregano, dried
1$^{1}/_{4}$ cups cooked dried beans (cannellini)

Method

- Put all ingredients except beans in a large saucepan and bring to boil.
- Reduce heat and simmer for 1 hour.
- Add beans.
- Take out three cups of soup, puree in a blender, then return to pot.
- Stir well, heat and serve.

Nutritional analysis per serve

Vitamin E
Age 1–3 years: 0.5 mg ATE—10% RDI
Age 4–7 years: 0.5 mg ATE— 8% RDI
Age 8–11 years: 0.5 mg ATE— 6% RDI

Vitamin C
For all children: 15 mg—50% RDI

Selenium
For all children: 126 mg—approx. 280% RDI

Using two different-coloured melons makes this fruit plate more attractive to children.

Ingredients

Makes 1 serve

1/4 cup honeydew melon, diced

1/4 cup rockmelon, diced

Method

- Combine the melons and arrange on a plate.

Nutritional analysis per serve

Vitamin C
For children of all ages: 23 mg—77% RDI

Cocoa powder is very rich in antioxidants. Use it to flavour drinks and foods, and don't forget the old favourite, hot chocolate.

Ingredients

Makes 1 serve

2 teaspoons cocoa powder

250 ml milk, whole

2 teaspoons sugar

Method

- Place two teaspoons of cocoa in a cup
- Pour hot milk over the cocoa and stir.
- Add sugar and stir well.

Nutritional analysis per serve A rich source of flavonoids.

6
Probiotics: functional foods

Probiotics are living microbes that have a beneficial effect on health by improving the microbial balance in the intestine. Naturally present in fermented foods like sour milk (consumed in some European and Middle East cuisines), probiotics are now included in foods like yoghurt and fermented milk drinks. They form part of the family of 'functional foods'—foods that claim to have a positive effect on health.

To understand the role of probiotics in boosting the immune system we need to look briefly at the inner environment of your child's digestive tract. At birth, children have sterile digestive tracts but within hours they become colonised by bacteria. As soon as food enters the digestive tract it brings with it opportunistic microbes that are looking for a home. Most of these bacteria are what we affectionately call 'friendly bacteria' because they actually help to establish and maintain a healthy digestive tract. At times, however, harmful types of bacteria reach the intestines, causing infections such as gastroenteritis. The bacteria occupying the gut are together referred to as the *intestinal flora* or the *microflora.*

To protect itself against harmful microbes the digestive system has its own specialised defence force. This defence system is composed, first, of millions of epithelial cells that line the inside of the gut and act as a physical protective layer. In addition, there are specialised cell clusters called *Payer's patches* which signal the presence of unfriendly microbes and call on the fighter cells for help. The fighter cells come in large numbers and take up position on the surface of the digestive tract where they bombard the harmful microbes with antibodies, to prevent their entry from the gut into the bloodstream.

Scientists now think that the friendly bacteria that live in the digestive tract also help to prevent infection from harmful microbes. Let's look at how.

Probiotics and immunity of the gut

There are many proposed ways in which probiotics are able to strengthen the immune system and prevent infections. These beneficial functions of probiotics can be categorised into two health benefits: resistance against colonisation of harmful bacteria and stimulation of the immune system. Probiotics offer resistance against harmful bacteria by blocking their attachment to the cells lining the inside of the gut, as well as by producing a number of substances that are toxic to harmful bacteria. Just how they stimulate the immune system is not fully known, however a number of studies give evidence to that effect.

We have an estimated one hundred trillion bacteria living in our digestive tract and an estimated four hundred different bacterial communities in the gut, some beneficial and some harmful. The microflora are very dynamic, with both beneficial and harmful bacteria competing with each other on a continual basis. When colonised by friendly bacteria the microflora help to strengthen the immune system. Friendly bacteria form the first line of defence by physically attaching themselves to the surface of the gut. Once firmly latched on to the gut wall, they prevent harmful bacteria from taking a foothold and eventually making their entry into the bloodstream. Unable to hold on to the gut wall, the harmful bacteria are simply passed out of the intestine. There is also some evidence that probiotics can alter the epithelial cells to strengthen their effectiveness against invading organisms.

Some friendly bacteria have evolved a further tactic against their unfriendly competitors. They produce certain metabolites, or chemical signals, to mark their territories and deter other microbes from colonising the same space, much like animals protecting their territories. These substances are toxic to harmful bacteria.

Research suggests that the beneficial effects of friendly bacteria are not limited to their presence in the digestive tract. They are capable of enhancing the resistance of the immune system to dangerous microbes, boosting the fighting ability of immune cells in the bloodstream. The mechanism of these benefits is not yet fully known. Research with lactobacillus GG strain, for example, showed a faster immune response to rotavirus. Consumption of lactobacillus GG significantly reduced the duration of diarrhoea due to rotavirus infection.

When things get out of balance

The composition of the microflora is relatively constant, with friendly bacteria dominating the harmful types. There are, however, a number of factors that can upset this balance in children. The main causes of an imbalance in the microflora are:

- radical changes in the diet;
- ingestion of new bacteria;
- antibiotics;
- emotional stress.

The usual symptoms of an imbalance are transient diarrhoea and minor belly pains.

Probiotics

The living microbes that we call 'probiotics' have beneficial effects on health by improving the intestinal microbial balance. The most beneficial of these microbes are the lactic acid bacteria. The first clue to these beneficial actions of probiotics on the microflora came from a Russian scientist in 1907. Metchnikoff claimed that the inclusion of yoghurts and fermented milk drinks, like sour milk, in the diet had a beneficial effect because they contained a special type of bacteria called lactobacilli. Scientists now know that these friendly bacteria live in the digestive tract but in unfavourable conditions their numbers decline and must be replenished from oral sources. There are several types of lactobacilli and also other friendly bacteria called bifidobacteria. The most important of these two types are *Lactobacillus acidophilus* and *Bifidobacterium bifidum.*

There are many other friendly bacteria in the gut but not all make good probiotics because not all survive the journey through the intestinal tract. It is all very well to have friendly bacteria flexing their muscles in a laboratory container and being heralded as the next Mike Tyson against harmful microbes. This alone is not sufficient—the bacteria must first survive the journey through the digestive system and, most importantly, the passage through the stomach which with its acidic contents stops many microbes.

The selection criteria for a useful probiotic are:

- the ability to survive the digestive juices, and colonise the intestinal tract;
- the ability to compete with harmful bacteria—it must stand its ground once established in the intestinal tract;
- the ability to stimulate the immune system; and, finally and very importantly,

- It must store well in chilled and dried food preparations so that it can be used by the food industry.

Not all types of bacteria have all these four qualities, so some are more useful than others in protecting the microflora. Lactobacilli are the major useful probiotic organisms, with *Lactobacillus acidophilus* La1 and *Lactobacillus rhamnosus* GG strains being particularly helpful. When it comes to the ability to latch on to the gut wall, these bacteria are the best. *Lactobacillus acidophilus* La1 is able to knock out salmonella and listeria, which are very toxic organisms responsible for food poisoning, always looking for a chance to colonise the gut and to squeeze their way into the bloodstream. *Lactobacillus rhamnosus* GG produces antimicrobial substances effective against *E. coli, Streptococus, Salmonella* and *Clostridium* species.

A study published in the *Journal of Dairy Science* in 1995 looked at changes in the immune system after consumption of lactic acid bacteria. When drunk by healthy volunteers, fermented milk containing *Lactobacillus acidophilus* La1 strain invigorated a specific type of fighter cell swimming in the bloodstream to the extent that they gobbled up foreign invaders much faster than before. In addition, ingestion of La1 resulted in a faster and more powerful antibody response against *Salmonella typhi* bacterium.

Lactobacillus rhamnosus GG strain and *Lactobacillus casei* have been shown to be effective in the treatment of gastroenteritis, in particular the type caused by a rotavirus that is common in infants and very young children. In a group of infants receiving *L. rhamnosus* GG the levels of fighter cells and antibodies against the rotavirus increased and offered protection against reinfection. Another study in children aged 4–45 months, who were infected with the rotavirus, showed that those who consumed lactobacillus GG had a shorter duration of diarrhoea than the children who received a placebo. Eating lactobacillus GG shortened the duration of diarrhoea from 2.4 days to 1.4 days. Further evidence

Table 6.1

Examples of probiotics and their food sources in Australian supermarkets

Probiotic	Available in
L. acidophilus	Jalna Bio Garde Swiss vanilla drinking yoghurt
	Nestle LC1 vanilla yoghurt
	Vaalia French vanilla drink and reduced fat yoghurt
	Bornhoffen natural yoghurt
	Yoplus Light 100% natural reduced fat yoghurt
	Bulla AB strawberry reduced fat drinking yoghurt*
L. casei	Bios fermented milk drink**
	Yakult
L. rhamnosus GG	Vaalia French vanilla drink and reduced fat yoghurt
Bifidobacteria	Vaalia French vanilla drink and reduced fat yoghurt
	Yoplus Light 100% natural reduced fat yoghurt
	Danone BIO

* An investigation by the Australian Consumer Association into the bacteria survival of probiotics available in Australian supermarkets in September 1999 found that this product has less than the optimal amount of *L. acidophilus.*

** An investigation by the Australian Consumer Association into the bacteria survival of probiotics available in Australian supermarkets in September 1999 found that near the end of this product's shelf life, the level of *L. casei* is insufficient to have beneficial effects.

of the benefits of consuming *Lactobacillus rhamnosus* GG to shorten the duration of diarrhoea came from a trial in children with acute diarrhoea in 1998. The duration of all types of diarrhoea (including diarrhoea caused by rotavirus) was significantly reduced (on average from 72 to 58 hours).

A relatively new strain of lactobacilli bacteria, now available in supermarkets, goes by the name of *Lactobacillus reuteri.* This friendly bacterium produces an antimicrobial substance called reuterin which can reduce the levels of harmful bacteria like salmonella and listeria in the intestine. For sources of probiotics in Australian supermarkets, see Table 6.1.

In summary, there is reasonable evidence to suggest that probiotics are a useful addition in the treatment of gastroenteritis due to bacteria and viruses, with some reports also suggesting protection against yeast infections and *Helicobacter pylori* infections. Well designed studies are missing, however, to prove the usefulness of probiotics in the prevention of yeast and *Helicobacter pylori* infections.

Antibiotic use

Probiotics may be particularly helpful when children have bacterial infections requiring antibiotic treatment because antibiotics kill the friendly as well as the harmful types of bacteria. It is not uncommon for children to get colicky pain and diarrhoea following, or during, a course of antibiotics. These may be signs of an imbalance in the microflora. To help maintain a healthy balance and return the friendly bacteria to the digestive tract, probiotics may be given to children while they are on antibiotics. Eating food containing probiotics during the treatment, and also for a few weeks afterwards, will continue to return friendly bacteria to the intestinal flora and prevent reinfection.

We'll now take a look at what foods were found to contain probiotics in sufficient numbers to have immunity-boosting effects. A survey carried out by the Australian consumer magazine, *Choice,* in September 1999 found that Vaalia, Yoplus Light and Nestle LCI had consistently high levels of friendly bacteria. In the yoghurts, Vaalia French vanilla reduced fat yoghurt had sufficient amounts of *L. acidophilus* and *L. rhamnosus* GG, while Yoplus had sufficient amounts of *L. acidophilus* and bifidobacteria, and Nestle had sufficient amounts of *L. acidophilus.* In the fermented milk drinks available, Yakult and Bios had good content of *L. casei,* with Yakult's friendly bacteria surviving in sufficient numbers towards the end of the drink's shelf life.

If your child does not like yoghurt or fermented drinks there is another option you can explore to introduce probiotics into your child's diet—probiotics in powdered form. This can be mixed into drinks for children, with some being suitable from 12 months of age. Some of these powders do contain milk solids, however, and may not be suitable for children who have diarrhoea. A note on storing products in a powder form: once opened they should be stored in a dark glass container and kept in the refrigerator.

Probiotics in tablet form are the choice for children who are recovering from diarrhoea, and can't tolerate milk or other dairy products. It is a good idea to give children a course of probiotics in a tablet for a few weeks after diarrhoea to help reestablish healthy microflora. The tablets are usually in a chewable form. Probiotics in tablet forms are readily available in pharmacies. Remember to check for the appropriate dosage and age recommendations for each supplement. A daily intake of 10^9–10^{10} of viable organisms is sufficient.

Safety concerns

Are probiotics completely safe? After all, they are live bacteria. It seems there is no 'zero risk' when it comes to bacteria but so far there have been no reports to suggest that there are health risks associated with giving probiotics to healthy children.

There have been no reported cases of clinical infection caused by consuming probiotic lactic acid bacteria, and no reports of deleterious metabolic or toxic effects.

Another concern is the possibility of 'gene hopping'—the transfer of genetic codes between probiotics and naturally occurring bacteria in the gut. This issue has implications for the future if genetically modified probiotics are allowed into supermarkets. Genetically modified yeast and bacteria already exist in the laboratory, engineered to withstand the degradation of enzymes as well as the more acidic conditions of the stomach. Work is being carried out to make them more resistant to antibiotics. Although beneficial in aim, this type of research carries with it potential risks. At present, to the best of my knowledge, no genetically engineered bacteria culture has been used in the probiotics found in Australian supermarkets.

Easy ways to introduce probiotics into children's diets

- Use yoghurt containing *L. acidophilus, L. casei, L. rhamnosus* GG of bifidobacteria in place of, or as an addition to, ice-cream when making fruit smoothies.
- Add small amounts of plain yoghurt (see above) to thicken soups (e.g. pumpkin), mild curries and baked potatoes.
- Alternatively, use powdered forms of probiotics to mix into fruit smoothies and other milk drinks.

7

Vegetarian diets and the immune system

A vegetarian diet includes a variety of foods from all the five food groups, as does a non-vegetarian diet, with the main difference being in the *type of protein foods* chosen from the Meat and Alternatives group. There are varying degrees of vegetarianism, depending on the amount of animal products omitted from the diet. The two main groups are known as total vegetarians or *vegans*, and *lacto-ovo-vegetarians*. Vegans abstain from all animal products, including meat, poultry, seafood, dairy products and eggs. Lacto-ovo-vegetarians avoid only meats, poultry and seafood, and include dairy products and eggs in their diets.

A well balanced, lacto-ovo-vegetarian diet can meet the nutritional needs of children, and can be planned to include adequate amounts of the nutrients that are important in boosting the immune system. Lack of variety and inadequate planning of meals, however, can place children at risk of poor nutrition, with the immune-boosting nutrients iron and zinc, as well as protein, in short supply. On the other hand, a lacto-ovo-vegetarian diet is rich in fruit and vegetables which supply children with plentiful amounts of vitamin C and antioxidant nutrients. If nuts and seeds as well as vegetables form a regular part of the diet, vitamin E needs are easily met.

Let's look at the strengths and weaknesses of the main types of vegetarian diets in more detail, and consider how to overcome the weaknesses of a vegetarian diet in boosting a child's immunity.

Vegetarian diets: strengths and weaknesses

Let's consider the two main types of vegetarian diets and see how each fares for its content of immune-boosting nutrients. When looking at the diets we must consider not only the actual content of the nutrient in the diet but also the ease with which children can digest and absorb the nutrients from plant sources.

We'll begin with a *lacto-ovo-vegetarian* diet. This is a diet based on breads and cereals, fruit and vegetables, and includes legumes, seeds and nuts, dairy products and eggs. Table 7.1 sets out the details of the nutrients available.

Now let's look at the *vegan* diet and how it meets the nutrient needs of children. A vegan diet is composed only of foods derived from plants, and includes grains, legumes, nuts, seeds, fruit and vegetables. Table 7.2 presents the details.

Table 7.1

The strengths and weaknesses of a lacto-ovo-vegetarian diet in childhood

Immunity-boosting nutrient	Adequate	May be low	At high risk
Protein	✔		
Kilojoules	✔		
Vitamin A	✔		
Iron		✔	
Zinc		✔	
Antioxidants	✔		
Probiotics	✔		

Table 7.2

The strengths and weaknesses of a vegan diet in childhood

Immunity-boosting nutrient	Adequate	May be low	At high risk
Protein			✔
Kilojoules			✔
Vitamin A		✔*	
Iron			✔
Zinc			✔
Antioxidants	✔		
Probiotics			✔

* A vegan diet, being rich in fruit and vegetables, is usually high in provitamin A, which turns into vitamin A once inside the body.

A quick glance at Table 7.2 shows that almost all nutrients important to building healthy immunity are likely to be in short supply in a vegan diet. A vegan diet is bulky and filling and children may feel 'full' before they have eaten adequate kilojoules. The vegan diet is unlikely to provide sufficient amounts of nutrients, particularly iron and protein important for a robust immunity. In addition, absorption of zinc and iron is poorer from plant foods. Because of these weaknesses the vegan diet is not suitable to boost children's immunity. From now on we consider only the lacto-ovo-vegetarian diet.

The lacto-ovo-vegetarian diet

Protein

We'll consider first the main sources of *protein* in a lacto-ovo-vegetarian diet. In addition to dairy products and eggs, which supply animal-derived proteins, the other sources of protein in the lacto-ovo-vegetarian diet are nuts, seeds and legumes. Nuts are high in protein—walnuts, for example, contain 28% of protein in comparison to beef, which has 22%. Legumes, which are very versatile in cooking, are also rich sources of protein, with soybeans

Sources of protein in a lacto-ovo-vegetarian diet for children over 12 months

- Milk, yoghurt and cheese (except cream cheese)
- Eggs
- Ground nuts: almond meal, macadamia, pecans, walnuts, carob flour
- Nut butters, e.g. almond butter
- Legumes: black-eyed beans, peas, chickpeas, lentils, lima beans, soybeans, peanuts
- Tofu (soybeans)
- Soy drink and soy yoghurts
- Seeds: sunflower, sesame (ground or as a paste, e.g. tahini)

being the best. However, despite their high protein content, all plant proteins, with the exception of soy, are of limited value for your child unless they are combined into well balanced meals.

There are two reasons why a lacto-ovo-vegetarian diet needs more care with meal planning if it is to provide children with adequate amounts of protein. First, the digestibility of proteins found in plant foods is lower than the digestibility of muscle proteins. For example, diets based on wholegrains, legumes and vegetables have a lower protein digestibility of 75–85%, while typical mixed diets including refined cereals and meats have a protein digestibility of 95%. An easy way of thinking about protein digestibility is as a measure of how much protein will be absorbed from the protein-containing foods. The better the protein digestibility the more protein will be absorbed into the body. Vegetarian diets, in comparison with a mixed diet that includes meat muscle, have a lower protein digestibility. This is due mostly to the presence of natural plant chemicals that interfere with protein absorption.

A lacto-ovo-vegetarian diet, which usually derives about half its protein from dairy products and eggs, needs no extra protein allowances, however. As long as children are consuming dairy products in the recommended amounts for their age, and eggs are a regular part of their diet, their need for protein is the same as for children eating a mixed diet that includes meat. The recommendations for protein in Chapter I are just as relevant to children on a lacto-ovo-vegetarian diet as they are for children consuming an omnivore's diet.

Second, unlike animal foods, plant foods don't contain all the essential amino acids that are necessary not only for a healthy immune system but also for normal growth and development. Plant proteins are low in one or two specific essential amino acids. The Protein Digestibility Corrected Amino Acid Scores (PDCAAS) offer a means to rate protein-rich foods according to their nutritional usefulness. The World Health Organization and the Food and Agriculture Organization of the United Nations have adopted the PDCAAS as the best system available for evaluating proteins. According to this system, the best quality proteins—that is, proteins that contain the best balance of essential amino acids—are found in milk (with a PDCAAS of 121) followed closely by those in eggs (PDCAAS of 118). Beef and soy proteins are ranked very closely together with a PDCAAS of 92 and 91 respectively. Soy protein shows the best amino acid composition by far of all plant foods; most plant proteins, have a significantly lower PDCAAS (wheat, for example, has a PDCAAS of 42). Soy drinks and tofu increase the relative protein quality of a vegetarian diet.

Despite poorer ratings in their ability to provide good quality protein, plant foods may be combined together to achieve vegetarian meals with complete sets of the essential amino acids. For example, cereals are low in lysine and threonine, while legumes are low in methionine and cysteine. When a cereal such as wheat is combined with a legume such as split pea, the combined pair share a complete set of amino acids between them.

Recent research suggests, however, that diets relying solely on complementary pairing of plant proteins to provide children with essential amino acids are inferior to diets that include animal proteins. It appears that while the entire set of amino acids is achieved by combining specific plant foods together, the bioavailability of the essential amino acids is inferior, and less of the essential amino acids are absorbed. The addition of milk or eggs to a plant-based diet overcomes these shortcomings. Average protein intakes of children on lacto-ovo-vegetarian diets generally meet or exceed childhood recommendations.

Planning complete-protein vegetarian meals

Our aim is to plan meals that supply *complete proteins at each mealtime.* You will recall that complete proteins are proteins that have the entire set of amino acids, including all the essential amino acids. Essential amino acids are those that a child's body cannot make for itself but needs a steady supply from the diet. Plant proteins are limited in one or two essential amino acids. The absent amino acids in plant proteins differ between different plant foods. In combining vegetarian proteins we try to complement each protein by the addition of another.

Combining cereal grains and dried beans, for example, improves the overall balance of amino acids so that the meal supplies all the essential amino acids necessary for good health. This type of food combining to achieve complete proteins is called 'protein complementation' and can be accomplished with other combinations of plant proteins. Various plant groups complement each other, allowing us to supply children with the correct set of essential amino acids.

It is quite simple to remember how to achieve the right combinations for a balanced meal. These are the complementary pairs:

- grains and legumes, e.g. baked beans on toast;
- grains and seeds or nuts, e.g. breakfast cereal including nuts or

seeds (be careful with young children as they may choke on small nuts and seeds);
- vegetables with nuts and seeds, e.g. celery sticks with peanut butter;
- vegetables with legumes, e.g. a bean and vegetable hotpot.

Kilojoules

It is essential that children consume enough kilojoules to prevent protein wastage. If insufficient kilojoules are consumed, even a good amount of quality protein in the diet will not prevent wastage of amino acids, which will be changed into glucose for energy. In addition, fats—the principal sources of kilojoules in all diets—are carriers for the fat-soluble vitamins, vitamin A and vitamin E. Both are essential for a healthy immune system. The restriction of fats in children on a lacto-ovo-vegetarian diet may result in a poor intake of kilojoules as well as of vitamins A and E. However, surveys carried out on children who eat a lacto-ovo-vegetarian diet show that their growth rates are no lower than those of children who eat meat.

It is important to remember, however, that the lacto-ovo-vegetarian diet has a lower kilojoule density than a mixed diet. This generally means that children on a lacto-ovo-vegetarian diet need to eat more in order to obtain the same amount of kilojoules. Lack of kilojoules is not normally a problem, however, with the use of vegetable oils and spreads, full-cream dairy products and eggs, as well as nuts and seeds. It can become a problem if fats are overly restricted. Elimination of spreads and oils, nuts and seeds from young children's diets is unwise, as it places children at risk of consuming insufficient kilojoules and fat-soluble vitamins, with deleterious effects on their immunity and overall development.

For older children and, in some cases, young children, fats, particularly saturated fats, may be limited if the child is gaining weight too rapidly or is overweight. Seek help from an accredited dietitian or your local doctor if you are concerned about your child's weight.

Vitamin A

Due to the higher content of fruits and vegetables a vegetarian diet is high in provitamin A. Provitamin A refers to carotenoids, a group of molecules which, once absorbed, are chemically altered and become fully functional vitamin A. There are about 600 carotenoids with 50 able to be converted to vitamin A once absorbed. Beta carotene is of most value, and is found in dark yellow and orange-coloured fruits as well as dark leafy vegetables. Recent research shows that beta carotene is somewhat better absorbed from yellow and orange-coloured fruits and vegetables, and not so well from dark green leafy vegetables.

In addition to the carotenoids present in plant foods, the lacto-ovo-vegetarian diet supplies children with dairy products, which are a good source of vitamin A. Deficiency of vitamin A is unlikely in children who eat a balanced vegetarian diet.

Iron

Children aged between six months and twenty-four months are particularly vulnerable to iron deficiency. Iron is essential for the healthy growth and development of children, and those who lack iron come down with infections more frequently. Children who are exclusively breast-fed rely on iron sources in the mother's milk for an adequate supply. When later weaning onto solid foods, good food sources of iron become important. Iron in food is found in two forms: *haem* iron is found in liver, kidneys and lean red meat, poultry and seafood, while *non-haem* iron is found in legumes, egg yolks, wholemeal breads, wholegrain cereals, green leafy vegetables, nuts and seeds. There is some non-haem iron in muscle proteins but there is no haem iron in plant foods. Haem iron is well absorbed by the body, while non-haem iron is absorbed rather poorly. Less than 5% of non-haem iron is absorbed compared with 10–25% in meat muscle. Therefore, although plant sources contain relatively high amounts of non-haem iron, this type of iron is not well absorbed. Children who rely on non-haem iron foods to supply them with their iron must eat more iron-rich foods than children who eat foods rich in haem iron. To prevent iron deficiency, vegeterian meals for children should include good amounts of non-haem iron-rich foods often.

Some studies show that children on lacto-ovo-vegetarian diets eat an equivalent amount of iron to children eating a mixed diet that includes meat. But, considering the poorer absorption of non-haem iron found in plant sources, this does not seem enough to guarantee prevention of iron deficiency. The World Health Organization estimates that 10–15% of iron is absorbed from diets in most industralised countries, including Australia, while absorption of iron from a vegetarian diet excluding meat is about 8%. Based on these figures, children on vegetarian diets must consume more iron than children on mixed diets including meat. Putting it another way, if a lacto-ovo-vegetarian diet contains comparable amounts of iron to a mixed diet, the lacto-ovo-vegetarian diet supplies less useful iron. So a vegetarian diet must be planned carefully to meet children's iron needs.

Providing vitamin C with meals can increase the absorption of non-haem iron. By including vegetables that are good sources of vitamin C, or offering citrus fruit just after the meal, the overall non-haem iron absorption can be increased by up to four times. To achieve these benefits the vitamin C and iron is best consumed at the same meal. Recent research shows that citric acid, which is plentiful in citrus fruit, enhances the absorption of iron in addition to vitamin C, so serving citrus fruit or diluted citrus fruit juice will further increase the absorption of non-haem iron.

Iron absorption can be inhibited by phytic acid which is present in wholegrains and legumes. Refined grains are much lower in phytates than wholegrain cereals, but the iron content of wholegrain cereals is higher than that of refined cereals, so the higher content of wholegrain cereals compensates for the poorer absorption. In addition, yeast breaks down the structure of phytates and improves the absorption of iron from baked products such as bread. Addition of vitamin C to a meal containing legumes (e.g. dried beans, lentils, peas) also helps to counteract the inhibiting effects of phytates on iron absorption.

Tannins in tea and cocoa reduce the absorption of non-haem iron by half. This is easily avoided by not serving tea to children at mealtimes. In addition, calcium in dairy products can markedly reduce iron absorption, so avoid mixing food sources high in calcium and iron in the one meal.

To improve iron absorption from a meal:

- Offer diluted fruit juice, or citrus fruit, with or after meals.
- Include vegetables rich in vitamin C as part of a meal.
- Avoid serving tea, cocoa or milk with meals rich in iron.
- Avoid offering cola.

Sources of iron in a lacto-ovo-vegetarian diet

Good sources of iron in a lacto-ovo-vegetarian diet are green leafy vegetables, wheat germ, wholegrain cereals, wholemeal breads, nuts, dried peas and beans, lentils, prunes, dates and apricots. Table 7.3 gives details.

Zinc

Zinc is essential for a healthy immune system in children and, if your child is eating within the guidelines of a lacto-ovo-vegetarian diet, then you must take extra care to ensure an adequate supply of zinc in your child's diet. Zinc is relatively hard to obtain in adequate amounts from diets that exclude lean meats and seafood,

Table 7.3

Iron content of foods in a lacto-ovo-vegetarian diet

Food	Portion	Amount (mg)*
Bread and cereals		
Bread, white	24 g	0.3
Bread, wholemeal	24 g	0.5
Breakfast cereal	28 g	2.4
Oats	1/2 cup	0.7
Pearl barley	1/2 cup	1.0
Rice, brown	1/2 cup	0.5
Rice, white	1/2 cup	0.3
Wheat germ	1 tbsp	0.6
Fruit and vegetables		
Avocado, raw	40 g	0.3
Baked beans	1/4 cup	1.1
Broccoli, cooked	45 g	0.5
Brussels sprouts	1/4 cup	0.6
Chickpeas	1/4 cup	2.8
Lentils	1/4 cup	0.9
Peas	1/4 cup	0.5
Prunes	40 g	0.5
Prunes, stewed	40 g	0.1
Pumpkin, boiled	1/4 cup	0.3
Raisins	25 g	1.1
Soybeans	1/4 cup	0.9
Spinach, English, cooked	1/4 cup	1.1
Meat alternatives (raw)		
Bean curd (tofu)	40 g	3.2
Cashews	15 g	0.8
Egg	45 g	0.7
Molasses	1 tsp	0.3
Pumpkin seeds	15 g	1.5
Sunflower seeds	15 g	0.7
Tahini, sesame butter	15 g	0.8
Walnuts	15 g	0.4

* RDI for all children is 6–8 mg daily.
Source: FoodWorks Professional Edition, Copyright 1998–2000 Xyris Software.

zinc's best sources. In addition, zinc is not well absorbed from plant sources due to the presence of phytic acid and fibre. Phytates are dietary constituents that bind to zinc and prevent its absorption. Phytates are high in a typical vegetarian diet, and are found in foods that are good sources of zinc, for example, wholegrains and legumes. Hence, zinc in a vegetarian diet comes packaged with phytates, which reduces its absorption (with the exceptions of eggs and dairy products—these don't contain phytates and are regularly included in lacto-ovo-vegetarian diets).

Unlike with iron, vitamin C does not increase the absorption of zinc. The way we prepare foods, however, does make a difference to zinc's availability for absorption. By cooking legumes thoroughly we reduce the phytates' ability to bind zinc and so more zinc is absorbed. Bran, which is particularly high in phytates, should not be given to small children. For older children, add some bran to the baking mixture of muffins, fruit breads and fruit cakes.

Nuts and wheat germ are two very good sources of zinc in a lacto-ovo-vegetarian diet and should be used often and in many ways to increase the zinc content in your child's diet. The best sources of zinc in a lacto-ovo-vegetarian diet are legumes, eggs, milk and leafy vegetables.

The absorption of zinc from dairy foods is more efficient than from plant sources. But the calcium present in dairy foods joins hands with phytates and further inhibits the absorption of zinc from plant foods. So, avoid serving dairy products with plant foods rich in zinc.

To improve zinc absorption from a lacto-ovo-vegetarian diet:

- Avoid serving tea, cocoa or milk at mealtimes.
- Avoid sprinkling raw bran on cereals.
- Bran may be added to baking mixtures for older children.
- Cook legumes well until very soft.

Studies show that a lacto-ovo-vegetarian diet provides a similar amount of zinc to a typical mixed diet that includes meat. But, like iron, the absorption of zinc is significantly lower from plant sources, so meals rich in zinc must be a priority when planning main meals for children on lacto-ovo-vegetarian diets. The recipe section at the end of this chapter has nutritious, high-zinc meal and snack ideas. Table 7.4 shows the zinc content of foods in a lacto-ovo-vegetarian diet.

Antioxidant vitamins and flavonoids

A well balanced vegetarian diet is plentiful in fruit and vegetables, including citrus fruit, so it is rich in vitamin C. Studies show that vegetarians have a higher intake of vitamin C than omnivores. Vitamin E is not a problem either as many vegetables, as well as nuts and seeds, are great sources of vitamin E. For children under the age of 5 years, nuts and seeds should be ground and added to desserts, yoghurt and baking products. The vitamin E content of a vegetarian diet is relatively higher than in a typical mixed diet. Flavonoids are also plentiful, again due to the high content of fruits, vegetables and legumes.

Selenium

The amount of selenium in plant foods varies greatly depending on the soil content where the food was grown, while meats and other foods of animal origin don't differ significantly in their selenium content. Vegetarian children are potentially more at risk of selenium deficiency as their diets rely on plants being grown in soils with an adequate selenium content. Vegetarian children living in areas with soils poor in selenium must be offered foods typically high in selenium more often to prevent selenium deficiency. Lacto-ovo-vegetarian children, however, are guarded by the inclusion of dairy products and eggs in their diet. In areas with soils adequate in selenium there is no risk of selenium deficiency in a vegetarian diet (more on this in Chapter 9).

Table 7.4

Zinc content of foods in a lacto-ovo-vegetarian diet

Food	Portion	Amount (mg)*
Bread and cereals		
Millet	1/2 cup	0.6
Oats	1/2 cup	0.4
Pearl barley	1/2 cup	0.4
Puffed rice cereal	1/2 cup	0.2
Wheat germ	1 tbsp	0.5
Vegetables (cooked)		
Asparagus	1/4 cup	0.1
Beans, Lima, dry	1/4 cup	0.4
Beans, red	1/4 cup	0.5
Broccoli	1/4 cup	0.2
Chickpeas, dry	1/4 cup	0.5
Corn	1/4 cup	0.3
Lentils, dry	1/4 cup	0.4
Okra	1/4 cup	0.3
Peas	1/4 cup	0.3
Soybeans, dry	1/4 cup	0.7
Seaweed, raw	1/4 cup	0.3
Spinach, English	1/4 cup	0.2
Meat alternatives (raw)		
Bean curd (tofu)	1/4 cup	0.5
Brazil nuts	1 tbsp	0.5
Cashews, dry roasted	1 tbsp	0.7
Cheese, cheddar	30 g	1.1
Egg	45 g	0.4
Milk, fluid, whole	1/2 cup	0.5
Peanut butter	1 tbsp	0.7
Pumpkin seeds	1 tbsp	0.7
Sunflower seeds	1 tbsp	0.8
Tahini, sesame butter	1 tbsp	1.0
Yoghurt	100 g	0.5

* RDI for children 1–3 years is 4.5 mg; for children 4–7 years 6 mg and for children 8–11 years 9 mg.
Source: FoodWorks Professional Edition, Copyright 1998–2000 Xyris Software.

Copper

Studies show that a lacto-ovo-vegetarian diet provides slightly more copper than a typical mixed diet that includes meat. It is probably safe to say that copper deficiency is unlikely in a well balanced, lacto-ovo-vegetarian diet despite the slightly poorer absorption of copper from plant foods. Children eating a varied lacto-ovo-vegetarian diet that includes good sources of copper are at no risk of copper deficiency.

Probiotics

As the lacto-ovo-vegetarian diet includes dairy products, it doesn't restrict the provision of probiotics to children in any way. Yoghurt and probiotic drinks of all types are well within the guidelines of the lacto-ovo-vegetarian diet. For more information on probiotics and their role in immunity, refer to Chapter 6.

Serving hints for legumes and vegetables

Some children may dislike many vegetables and legumes. As both are important sources of nutrients in a vegetarian diet it is essential that a good variety of both is eaten. These hints will help to get your children interested in eating vegetables and legumes—remember to make the food interesting and simple to eat.

- Young children like finger food, so serve tofu in strips braised in a little sauce.
- Strips of steamed vegetables go down well (e.g. carrots, celery, zucchini).
- Puree some tofu into a cheese sauce and serve with macaroni.
- Blend avocado with cottage cheese and serve on bread or toast.
- Finely chopped vegetables can be added to spaghetti sauce or casseroles.

- Well-cooked legumes can be added to sauces.
- Chickpeas can be made into a paste called hummus, or you can purchase ready-made hummus from some food outlets and most health food stores. Serve with strips of vegetables or toast.
- Vegetables can be blended into soups for young children.

Cooking legumes

Legumes require soaking prior to cooking, with the exceptions of split peas, lentils and mung beans. Follow these steps for well cooked legumes.

Step 1 Rinse beans well, removing grit and discoloured beans.

Step 2 Cover beans with 3–4 times their volume of water and soak for about 12 hours. Place legumes in the refrigerator while soaking.

Step 3 Pour out the soak water and cook beans in fresh water. This improves digestion. Bring to the boil, then simmer partly covered, using Table 7.5 as a guide to cooking times.

Table 7.5

Cooking time for legumes

Legume	Ratio of legumes to water	Cooking time (hours)
Chickpeas	1 : 4	2–3
Kidney beans*	1 : 3.5	1–2
Lentils	1 : 3	0.5
Soybeans	1 : 4	2–3
Split peas	1 : 3	0.5

* Kidney beans contain a poison which is completely destroyed by adequate cooking. The method described above is safe, but avoid cooking beans slowly at low temperatures (less than 80°C), for example, in a crockpot, as lower temperatures do not destroy the poison.

This recipe is a great source of protein, zinc and iron, all of which can be in low supply in a vegetarian diet. It is also rich in vitamin A.

Ingredients

Makes approximately:
6 serves for 1–3 year olds
5 serves for 4–7 year olds
4 serves for 8–11 year olds

90 g split red lentils
1 cup water
1 medium onion, thinly sliced or chopped
10 ml olive oil
½ cup strong-flavoured cheddar cheese, grated
¼ cup dry cracked wheat
5 ml dried mixed herbs
1 large tomato, roughly chopped
1 tablespoon tomato puree

Method

- Wash the lentils in a sieve under the tap, removing any black ones.
- Bring to boil in the water and simmer, covered, for 15–20 minutes.
- Check occasionally, adding more water if the mixture is too dry. All the liquid should have been absorbed, leaving the lentils moist and soft, by the end of cooking time.
- Heat the oven to 180°C.
- While the lentils are cooking, brown the onion in the oil.
- Mix the onion, grated cheese, cracked wheat and herbs together.
- Add the lentils (draining off any excess fluid), tomatoes and the tomato puree.
- Tip the mixture into a greased shallow baking tin about 18 cm in diameter and bake for about 30 minutes until sizzling.

Nutritional analysis per serve

Protein
Age 1–3 years: 8 g—40% RDI
Age 4–7 years: 9 g—38% RDI
Age 8–11 years: 11 g—30% RDI

Zinc
Age 1–3 years: 1.0 mg—23% RDI
Age 4–7 years: 1.3 mg—21% RDI
Age 8–11 years: 1.6 mg—18% RDI

Iron
Age 1–3 years: 1.5 mg—22% RDI
Age 4–7 years: 1.8 mg—25% RDI
Age 8–11 years: 2.2 mg—32% RDI

For young children omit corn kernels and raisins. Use creamed corn and half a cup of grated apple drained of juice instead.

Ingredients

Makes approximately:
12 serves for 1–3 year olds
9 serves for 4–7 year olds
6 serves for 8–11 year olds

6 green capsicums
water
3 cups cooked basmati rice
1 cup cooked chickpeas
2 carrots, grated
1 cup whole-kernel corn
1/2 onion, chopped
1/2 cup raisins
1/2–1 cup grated mozzarella cheese
3–4 cups tomato sauce (see p. 116)
salt and freshly ground black pepper to taste

Method

- Cut the tops from the capsicums and discard seeds and membranes.
- Chop enough of the tops to make 1/4 cup, set aside.
- Fill a large pot about two-thirds full with water, bring to boil and cook whole capsicums for 5 minutes.
- Remove and invert to dry.
- In a large bowl, combine the remaining ingredients and reserved chopped capsicum.
- Preheat oven to 190°C.
- Cut capsicums in half lengthwise and stuff each half with the rice and chickpea mixture.
- Place the halves on a large baking tray.
- Bake for 30 minutes.
- Transfer peppers to a platter and serve warm.

Nutritional analysis per serve

Protein
Age 1–3 years: 10 g—50% RDI
Age 4–7 years: 13 g—55% RDI
Age 8–11 years: 20 g—55% RDI

Zinc
Age 1–3 years: 1.7 mg—40% RDI
Age 4–7 years: 2.3 mg—40% RDI
Age 8–11 years: 3.5 mg—40% RDI

Iron
Age 1–3 years: 2.8 mg—40% RDI
Age 4–7 years: 3.7 mg—50% RDI
Age 8–11 years: 5.6 mg—80% RDI

A quick way to introduce more nuts into your child's diet—nuts are a great source of protein, iron and zinc in a vegetarian diet.

Ingredients

Makes approximately 4 serves

125 g light cream cheese, or fresh ricotta cheese for older children

1/4 cup walnuts or pecans

1/4 cup chopped dried apricots

milk (optional)

Method

- Blend the nuts and apricots together in a blender.
- Mix nuts and apricots into the cheese—add some milk for a more runny consistency if desired.

Nutritional analysis per serve

Protein
Age 1–3 years: 4.4 g—25% RDI
Age 4–7 years: 4.4 g—10% RDI
Age 8–11 years: 4.4 g— 7% RDI

Iron
For all children: 0.5 mg—7% RDI

Zinc
Age 1–3 years: 0.5 mg—10% RDI
Age 4–7 years: 0.5 mg— 8% RDI
Age 8–11 years: 0.5 mg— 5% RDI

Spinach is by far the richest source of iron among vegetables. It is used with flair in this recipe.

Ingredients

Makes approximately:
10 serves for 1–3 year olds
8 serves for 4–7 year olds
6 serves for 8–11 year olds

2 medium onions, chopped

3 cloves garlic, minced

1 tablespoon olive oil

3 cups cooked chickpeas

1 package frozen chopped spinach, defrosted

1 x 880 g can crushed tomatoes

1 cup chopped fresh tomatoes

1 teaspoon crushed red capsicum flakes

1 teaspoon dried oregano

juice of 2 lemons

salt and black pepper to taste (omit for very young children)

Method

- Sauté the onions and garlic in the olive oil in a large saucepan over medium heat until the onions are tender.
- Add the chickpeas, spinach, tomatoes, pepper flakes and oregano.
- Cover and simmer for 30 minutes.
- Add the lemon juice, salt and pepper.

Nutritional analysis per serve

Protein
Age 1–3 years: 6.5 g—35% RDI
Age 4–7 years: 8.0 g—33% RDI
Age 8–11 years: 11.0 g—30% RDI

Iron
Age 1–3 years: 2.4 mg—34% RDI
Age 4–7 years: 3.0 mg—40% RDI
Age 8–11 years: 3.9 mg—55% RDI

Zinc
Age 1–3 years: 1.2 mg—35% RDI
Age 4–7 years: 1.5 mg—33% RDI
Age 8–11 years: 2.0 mg—30% RDI

Another great way to use spinach to increase iron in your child's diet. Most children love lasagne and they will enjoy this one. Serve with unsweetened diluted fruit juice or follow with fruit rich in vitamin C.

Ingredients

Makes approximately:
12 serves for 1–3 year olds
9 serves for 4–7 year olds
6 serves for 8–11 year olds

1 large bunch fresh spinach, stalks removed

250 g lasagne sheets

250 g fresh ricotta cheese

1 cup white sauce (see below)

2 tablespoons grated parmesan cheese

1¼ cups breadcrumbs

4 very ripe medium tomatoes, thinly sliced

1 medium onion, finely chopped

2 cloves garlic, finely chopped

1 tablespoon finely chopped fresh basil or 1 teaspoon dried basil

1 tablespoon finely chopped fresh oregano or 1 teaspoon dried oregano

2 tablespoons tomato paste, mixed with 1½ cups water or vegetable stock

freshly ground black pepper

1 teaspoon freshly grated nutmeg

White sauce

1 tablespoon monounsaturated margarine

3 teaspoons white flour

1 cup milk

Method

- Preheat oven to 200°C.
- In a large saucepan bring water to the boil.
- Drop in spinach leaves for 1 minute.
- Remove, drain well, chop finely and set aside.
- Bring a large saucepan of water to the boil, drop in lasagne sheets, 3 at a time.
- Cook for 10 to 12 minutes until tender.
- Plunge into cold water, drain and set aside.
- To make white sauce, melt margarine then add flour, mixing well to a smooth paste to make a roux. Cool. Bring milk to the boil then allow to cool for a few minutes. Gradually pour milk into the roux, mixing well with a wooden spoon to avoid lumps. If lumps form, pass through a fine strainer. Makes 1 cup.
- Mix ricotta and parmesan cheese with breadcrumbs until mixture is like crumbs, and divide into 4 portions.
- Layer a 30 cm x 20 cm non-stick baking dish in the following order:
  - 4 lasagne sheets
  - portion of breadcrumb mixture, followed by white sauce
  - spinach
  - tomatoes
  - onion and garlic
  - basil and oregano
- Repeat the process three times and top with a layer of lasagne sheets.
- Pour tomato paste and water mixture over the top.
- Sprinkle with remaining ricotta, parmesan and breadcrumb mixture.
- Season with pepper and sprinkle with nutmeg.
- Bake for 40 minutes until top is brown.

Nutritional analysis per serve

Protein
Age 1–3 years: 13 g—70% RDI
Age 4–7 years: 17 g—70% RDI
Age 8–11 years: 25 g—65% RDI

Zinc
Age 1–3 years: 1.1 mg—25% RDI
Age 4–7 years: 1.5 mg—25% RDI
Age 8–11 years: 2.2 mg—25% RDI

Iron
Age 1–3 years: 2.0 mg—30% RDI
Age 4–7 years: 2.7 mg—38% RDI
Age 8–11 years: 4.0 mg—57% RDI

Tofu picks up flavours wonderfully, as well as being a source of high-quality protein. Serve with fruit juice or follow the meal with fruit rich in vitamin C to increase iron absorption.

Ingredients

Makes 8 serves

350 g tofu

75 g breadcrumbs

1 large carrot, grated

1 onion, finely chopped

1 teaspoon fresh ginger root, grated finely

1 teaspoon dried mixed herbs

1½ tablespoons soy sauce, to taste

25 g wheat germ

Method

- Heat the oven to 190°C.
- Making sure the tofu is well drained, mix all the ingredients to a firm blend.
- Let the mixture stand for a few minutes.
- Shape into 8 burgers, and dip each one in the wheat germ.
- Bake on a greased tray for 15–20 minutes.
- Serve with tomato sauce mixed with smooth chilli sauce.

Nutritional analysis per serve

Protein
Age 1–3 years: 7.5 g—40% RDI
Age 4–7 years: 7.5 g—30% RDI
Age 8–11 years: 7.5 g—20% RDI

Iron
For all children: 4 mg—60% RDI

Zinc
Age 1–3 years: 0.9 mg—20% RDI
Age 4–7 years: 0.9 mg—15% RDI
Age 8–11 years: 0.9 mg—10% RDI

ASPARAGUS FRITTATA

Children love eggs and this egg dish is soft and yummy and rich in protein, vitamin A and zinc.

Ingredients

1 tablespoon olive oil

300 g small asparagus, thinly sliced

4 eggs, lightly beaten

100 ml full-cream milk

pepper

Makes approximately:
4 serves for 1–3 year olds
2 serves for older children

Method

- Heat the oil in a heavy-based frying pan and sauté the asparagus over a low heat for 10–15 minutes, or until soft.
- Mix the eggs, milk and pepper together and pour over asparagus.
- Cook until mixture is set underneath.
- Turn it over, or put the pan under a medium-hot grill for a few minutes, or until the frittata is golden and set.

Nutritional analysis per serve

Protein
Age 1–3 years: 10.5 g—60% RDI
Age 4–7 years: 21.0 g—55% RDI
Age 8–11 years: 21.0 g—55% RDI

Iron
Age 1–3 years: 1.7 mg—25% RDI
Age 4–7 years: 3.5 mg—50% RDI
Age 8–11 years: 3.5 mg—50% RDI

Zinc
Age 1–3 years: 0.8 mg—18% RDI
Age 4–7 years: 1.6 mg—18% RDI
Age 8–11 years: 1.6 mg—18% RDI

Ingredients

Makes 1 serve

½ cup cooked oats

1 tablespoon honey

1 tablespoon almond meal

125 ml milk

Method

- Cook the oats according to directions on packet, to make porridge.
- Mix in honey and almond meal.
- Pour milk over porridge.

Nutritional analysis per serve

Protein
Age 1–3 years: 8 g—40% RDI
Age 4–7 years: 8 g—30% RDI
Age 8–11 years: 8 g—20% RDI

Iron
For all children: 1.1 mg—16% RDI

Zinc
Age 1–3 years: 2 mg—44% RDI
Age 4–7 years: 2 mg—33% RDI
Age 8–11 years: 2 mg—22% RDI

For children under 5 years, substitute almond meal for sliced almonds and omit pine nuts.

Ingredients

Makes approximately 10 serves

100 g pitted prunes

40 g dried apricots

40 g dried figs

40 g raisins

2 tablespoons raw sugar

1 teaspoon rosewater

juice of 1/4 lemon

50 g roasted sliced almonds

20 g roasted pine nuts

Method

- Put fruit in large bowl.
- Sprinkle with sugar plus rosewater.
- Add water to cover.
- Stir to mix flavours.
- Cover with plastic wrap and leave to soak overnight.
- Transfer to saucepan, adding extra liquid to cover if needed.
- Bring to boil, then reduce heat and simmer for 10 minutes.
- Allow to cool slightly and stir in lemon juice to taste.
- Serve warm or chilled, sprinkled with nuts, with yoghurt on the side.

Nutritional analysis per serve

Protein
Age 1–3 years: 1.8 g—10% RDI
Age 4–7 years: 1.8 g— 8% RDI
Age 8–11 years: 1.8 g— 5% RDI

Iron
For all children: 0.7 mg—10% RDI

Zinc
Age 1–3 years: 0.4 mg—9% RDI
Age 4–7 years: 0.4 mg—7% RDI
Age 8–11 years: 0.4 mg—4% RDI

These potatoes are soft and flavoursome; topped with avocado stuffing they offer a meal rich in vitamin E as well as protein, zinc and iron.

Ingredients

Makes approximately:
3 serves for 1–3 year olds
1–2 serves for 4–7 year olds
1 serve for 8–11 year olds

3 small baking potatoes
oil and sea salt, for brushing

Avocado stuffing

½ cup avocado, diced
125 g cottage cheese
1 teaspoon onion, finely chopped
pinch of pepper
1 tablespoon lemon juice

Method

- Wash the potatoes, pat dry, prick with a fork, brush with oil and sprinkle with a little sea salt.
- Place in a preheated oven (190°C) and bake for about 40 minutes, or until crispy on the outside and tender inside (test with a skewer).
- Cut the potatoes in half, scoop out some of the flesh into a bowl and mash thoroughly.
- To make the avocado stuffing, mash the avocado and cheese together then add the finely chopped onion, pepper and lemon juice.
- Mix mashed potato with the avocado stuffing then spoon the mixture back into the scooped out skins.
- Place the potatoes under a preheated grill.
- Heat for a few minutes, until lightly golden on top.

Nutritional analysis per serve

Protein
Age 1–3 years: 9 g—50% RDI
Age 4–7 years: 13 g—60% RDI
Age 8–11 years: 27 g—70% RDI

Iron
Age 1–3 years: 0.8 mg—11% RDI
Age 4–7 years: 1.2 mg—17% RDI
Age 8–11 years: 2.4 mg—35% RDI

Zinc
Age 1–3 years: 0.7 mg—16% RDI
Age 4–7 years: 1.0 mg—17% RDI
Age 8–11 years: 2.1 mg—23% RDI

8

Feeding children during illness

Infection causes two major changes that are relevant to the provision of nutrition to children. First, there are physical symptoms that make eating more difficult and, second, there are increased requirements for some of the nutrients important in the fight against infection. We will look at these two in turn.

Nutrition priorities during colds, flu and gastroenteritis

'Mummy I don't feel like eating.' When children fall ill they often lose interest in food. This may be due to a sore throat, which makes swallowing food very difficult, or to a fever accompanied by a general loss of appetite. When children get a sore tummy, the situation becomes even more difficult. Should we be active in our attempt to feed children during illness, or should we take a more passive role? After all, it won't be long before they bounce back and regain their appetite.

To feed or not to feed?

It may be very difficult to tempt children with their usual foods but don't fall into the trap of offering treats just so that they eat something. Children are quick to take advantage of such situations—providing they don't have an upset tummy, they will ask for more of the same and refuse any other foods, making the most of your sympathy.

Maintaining the best possible nutrition during childhood illness is important for the following reasons:

- When fever is present, extra kilojoules are needed to prevent weight loss.
- When diarrhoea or vomiting sets in, extra fluid and electrolytes are needed to prevent dehydration.
- When your child is troubled by a sore throat this may last for some time and result in weight loss.
- During illness, the need for some vitamins and minerals increases as they are used up more quickly.

By looking after nutrition during illness we help to boost the immune system, which means faster recovery and less likelihood of recurrent infections.

Regardless of why your child is reluctant to eat, it is important that you continue to offer food and fluids often. The type of meals and snacks on offer may make a significant difference to the amount of food your child will actually eat. In the following sections we look at how to optimise your child's nutrition during sickness. We consider the most common symptoms and discuss the best feeding strategies for each.

Diarrhoea

The most common and most serious cause of diarrhoea in otherwise healthy children is gastroenteritis due to infection. The bugs responsible are most commonly viruses (e.g. rotavirus); less often, bacteria are the cause (e.g. salmonella) and sometimes protozoa (e.g. giardia lamblia).

The number one nutritional goal when caring for a child with diarrhoea (regardless of its cause) is to prevent or treat dehydration. The second priority is to provide nutrients called *electrolytes*—the two most important are potassium and sodium. Both fluid and electrolytes are lost in unusually high amounts during the course of diarrhoea, and must be replenished quickly. Remember that children dehydrate much more quickly than adults so they are more susceptible to the dangers of dehydration—these include fever, general malaise and, in severe cases, a life-threatening shutdown of vital organs.

Mild diarrhoea

To guard against the ill effects of dehydration from mild diarrheoa, it is most important to offer your child fluids often during the day and at night (unless your child is able to sleep and there is no diarrhoea). Fluid requirements are based on the weight of the child. Aim for 60–100 ml of fluid per half kilogram of body weight daily. Add extra for any fluid losses due to vomiting—estimate this amount as best you can. This is the daily fluid amount your child should drink until diarrhoea and vomiting settle.

A more practical guide is to offer your child a drink of 5–7 ml of fluid per kilogram of body weight every hour. For example, a 10 kilogram child would need 50–70 ml of fluid per hour (calculated on a 24-hour basis, giving fluids every two hours during the night, 100–150 ml each time). The choice of fluids depends on the child's age and preferences, but there are some drinks you should not offer. Don't give milk or milk products as they may worsen the diarrhoea. Milk contains lactose, a sugar that is not digested well during bouts of diarrhoea, as diarrhoeal illness temporarily damages the intestinal enzyme required for its digestion. Rehydrating is best done with clear fluids.

Full-strength fruit juice, cordial and soft drinks are unsuitable, however. Diluted fruit juices, weak tea sweetened with one teaspoon of sugar, and diluted cordial are all helpful. For young children, dilute fruit juice by using 50 ml unsweetened fruit juice and adding 200 ml of water. Dilute regular soft drink in the same ratio: one part soft drink to four parts water. Unlike water, these drinks contain some kilojoules, and so are helpful when your child is not eating well or is vomiting and cannot keep down solid food.

Ice blocks also count as fluid and these are usually very well liked. They may, however, worsen the diarrhoea if given in full strength as they are too concentrated. To prevent this, make your own ice blocks by freezing diluted cordial or fruit juices. This is easily done by freezing diluted juice or cordial in large ice cube trays and inserting ice-cream sticks just before they freeze. Children will often like to suck on these even if they are not making good progress with drinking fluids. For correct dilution of clear fluids, refer to Table 8.1.

Table 8.1

Correct dilution of clear fluids for diarrhoea and vomiting

Fluid	Dilution in water	Example
Oral rehydration solution	n/a	See directions on pack Mix with water only
Regular soft drink	1 part to 4 parts	20 ml soft drink with 80 ml water Use warm water to help get rid of the bubbles Suitable for freezing into ice blocks
100% fruit juice	1 part to 4 parts	20 ml juice to 80 ml water Suitable for freezing into ice blocks
Cordial concentrate	1 part to 20 parts	5 ml (1 tsp) cordial concentrate to 100 ml water Suitable for freezing into ice blocks

Sports drinks advertised for their ability to rehydrate athletes during physical activity are unsuitable for children with diarrhoea or vomiting. These are too high in sugar and too low in salt to be a suitable rehydration fluid for children.

Bonox and broth are savoury alternatives that can be drunk warm in winter. Homemade chicken soup helps to replenish lost salts and has a good amount of protein. Protein-rich foods are usually not popular with children who have poor appetites, but chicken soup is usually well liked and helps to provide much needed protein. If your child is not up to eating soup containing solid pieces of chicken and vegetables, strain the soup so there are no solids and offer the liquid to sip. This is much easier and it still contains all the goodies I mentioned above.

Commercial oral rehydration fluids are not necessary if your child has one or two small bouts of diarrhoea during the day, doesn't vomit and has a good intake of clear fluids as discussed above. Oral rehydration fluids are, however, essential for the treatment of more severe diarrhoea, with or without vomiting.

Severe diarrhoea

If diarrhoea is complicated by vomiting, or is particularly severe, then a commercial oral rehydration solution is needed as a source of fluid. Oral rehydrating solutions like Gastrolyte work more quickly to rehydrate children because they are absorbed more readily. They also contain sodium and potassium in the correct amounts to supply the body. Oral rehydrating solutions may be bought from a pharmacy without a prescription. Mix the powder very carefully to make sure it is fully dissolved.

The three steps to managing *acute* diarrhoea in children:

- Give oral rehydrating solution, e.g. Gastrolyte, on its own for four hours.

- Reintroduce a light diet and continue to offer solids if there is no nausea; otherwise, continue with fluids only.
- Continue to offer oral rehydrating solution and other suitable fluids for the duration of diarrhoea and/or vomiting.
- Introduce easily digestible (light) foods no later than 24 hours after vomiting stops, even if faeces is still loose.

Soluble fibre—which is the type found in fruit and vegetables as well as some grains—has been found helpful in reducing children's diarrhoea. If your child has diarrhoea but no upset tummy, you may want to try a diet high in soluble fibre, based mostly on rice, oats, peeled apples and ripe bananas.

Nausea and vomiting

Children will rarely want to eat or drink when vomiting as they are afraid it will make them vomit again. A break in their usual food intake is to be expected but do persist with drinks as they will need to rehydrate.

The clear fluids discussed in the section on managing diarrhoea are also helpful in managing vomiting. Children who feel nauseous will usually take a few small sips. These do not go far, and frequent sips are needed. Offer fluids as often as possible, at least every hour. Once nausea has subsided, larger volumes of liquid should be given with the aim of meeting the child's daily fluid requirements.

Do take children to see a doctor if they cannot meet their daily fluid needs. You should aim for 60–100 ml per half kilogram body weight daily, or 5–7 ml of fluid per kilogram body weight per hour.

Once clear fluids are well tolerated you may introduce foods that are easy on the tummy. Try toast, crackers or teething rusks

For children of all ages, seek medical advice if:

- diarrhoea is more serious than usual and goes on for more than 24 hours
- your child vomits frequently and cannot retain any fluids
- you notice signs of dehydration: sunken eyes, no tears, dry lips and mouth
- your child has not passed urine in the last 4–6 hours
- your child has tummy ache or a high fever

for small children. Then progress to chicken soup with rice or noodles, rice pudding or grated apple, slowly returning to their regular diet. Reintroducing milk must be done slowly. Once tolerated in small amounts, increase gradually to the usual amount. The following foods are suitable when recovering from nausea, vomiting or diarrhoea:

- bread or toast with a thin spread of butter/margarine and vegemite;
- rice and apples;
- refined cereals like puffed rice or cornflakes, dry, to snack on;
- cooked mashed potato, pumpkin or carrots;
- lean chicken, veal, pork or fish—small serves; may be better tolerated if given cold and sliced thinly;
- yoghurt, especially with probiotics;
- custard and ice-cream in moderation—avoid if diarrhoea is particularly severe or prolonged;
- soft, peeled fruit;
- soups.

Avoid fried, fatty, spicy and take-away foods for a few days.

Fever

During a fever the metabolic rate rises and causes a greater expenditure of energy. A feverish child will need extra kilojoules to maintain body weight. A useful rule of thumb is: for every degree rise in temperature, kilojoule needs rise by 7%. This is a significant increase: children who require 5800 kilojoules to maintain their weight in health may need to eat an extra 400 kilojoules to prevent weight loss. If the child's physical activity is reduced as a result of fever, the additional calories may not be necessary. To provide sufficient kilojoules daily children should be offered foods and nourishing fluids more often. Roughly every two hours is a good aim. Cool fluids and soft cool foods will be better tolerated than cooked hot foods.

Fluid requirements also increase during fever. Offer fluids frequently and encourage the child to drink as much as possible.

Upper respiratory illness

Sore throats, sniffles and sneezes don't add up to a good appetite. Nevertheless, children should be encouraged to eat as well as possible. When children have a cold, the sneezing, coughing and, in particular, the nose dripping causes greater fluid loss. To make up for this they must drink a little more. Warm soothing liquids are best. Broth, warm milk, weak tea with lemon and sugar or honey (for the older child) and real, homemade lemonade are well liked and help to soothe the symptoms temporarily. Fruit juice diluted by half with water is also suitable.

As a sore throat makes swallowing foods particularly uncomfortable, soft foods are much better tolerated. Don't force food on a child—you don't want to develop food dislikes that will last well into the future. Instead, offer soft foods more often. If solid foods are refused, offer fluids or very soft options like puddings, creamed rice, custard and soft or grated fruit. You'll find many helpful recipes at the end of this chapter.

Infections eat up immunity-boosting nutrients

In fighting infection the immune system uses up the stores of nutrients important to its function. Studies show that nutrients capable of acting as antioxidants are in higher demand during infections than during health. Vitamin E and zinc are used up at a faster rate in the process of controlling free radical damage. It is important to replace these nutrients to build up the store in the body. Low body stores result in a less efficient immune response, which may lead to prolonged or more severe infectious illness.

In the period just after an illness, the first few weeks are most crucial in restocking the nutrients important in boosting children's immunity. The diet in those few weeks should be carefully planned to include good amounts of these nutrients to help replenish your child's body stores.

Supplements

When children's appetites are low and they are not eating their usual amount of food, or will eat certain foods only, they may not be consuming an adequate variety of food. At such times, supplements may offer a helping hand. Look for a multivitamin formulated for children that includes a good mix of nutrients important in boosting immunity. Refer to Chapter 9 for further information on suitable supplements.

Getting your child to drink enough during illness can be tricky. Fruit juice pops are a good way to increase their fluid intake as most children like them even during nausea.

Ingredients

1 cup orange juice, freshly squeezed

1 cup water

Method

- Strain orange juice to remove pips.
- Combine juice with water.
- Pour the mixture into popsicle moulds.
- Insert ice-cream sticks after 1–1½ hours in the freezer.
- Freeze until hard, at least 2 hours.

Children who have sore throats find it difficult to eat fresh fruit, yet fresh fruit is the best source of vitamin C and other antioxidants. The following ways of preparing fruit ensure that the texture is suitable for even the sorest of throats.

Grated apple

Wash and peel a Granny Smith apple. Finely grate and drizzle with lemon juice. You may want to add caster sugar to taste. Other suitable fruits include bananas and pears.

Fruit juice

Pineapple, melons, oranges and apples are great to juice from fresh. Remember to dilute all juices half/half with water.

Raspberries make for the best flavour and the smoothest texture in this jelly.

Ingredients

Makes 4–6 serves

450 g berry fruits (raspberries, blackberries, blueberries, strawberries)

2 tablespoons arrowroot

150 ml water

3 tablespoons honey

Method

- In a saucepan, mix the arrowroot to a smooth paste with a little of the water.
- Whisk in the remaining water and add the fruit (except raspberries) and half the honey.
- Place saucepan on a medium heat and bring the mixture to the boil, stirring.
- Simmer for 5 minutes to soften the fruit. If using raspberries, add them to the pan only 30 seconds before the end of cooking.
- Remove the mixture from the heat, add honey and let it cool.
- Blend until smooth.
- Pour the jelly into a serving dish and leave for several hours, until cold and lightly set.

This soup is a great source of protein, soluble fibre and antioxidants, and tastes good too.

Ingredients

Makes 1–2 serves

1½ cups chicken stock

1 tablespoon rice

1 egg yolk

squeeze of lemon juice

Method

- Bring stock to the boil in a small pan, add rice, cover and cook until rice is tender, about 12 minutes.
- Just before serving, beat egg yolk and lemon juice together.
- Add a little of the hot soup, stir, then whisk this mixture back into the pan of hot soup.
- Remove from heat immediately and serve.

Serve with toast for a nutritious meal full of protein, vitamin A and antioxidants. Omit toast and serve fresh soft white bread for children with sore throats.

Ingredients

Makes approximately:
4 serves for 1–3 year olds
2–3 serves for older children

2 medium tomatoes, fresh

40 g olive oil or olive oil margarine

75 g cheddar cheese, grated

1 egg, well beaten

salt and pepper

Method

- Scald and peel the fresh tomatoes.
- Chop the tomatoes finely.
- Add oil or melt the margarine in a frying pan, and add the tomatoes.
- Cook on slow heat for a few minutes, stirring occasionally.
- Add the cheese so it melts and mixes into the softened tomatoes.
- Place four egg rings in a pan and spoon the tomato and cheese mixture in.
- Add some of the beaten egg into each ring and season to taste.
- Cook for 2–3 minutes and serve warm or cool. You can also use as a filling for sandwiches, rolls or baguettes.

Fresh garlic is high in allicin, a natural ingredient that helps to fight germs. Garlic bread is the best way to include fresh garlic in your child's diet.

Great for children with colds in winter who have a runny nose but not a sore throat. Can be dunked in chicken soup or milk for children with sore throats.

Ingredients

2 x 1.5 cm thick slices Italian bread

1 clove garlic, peeled

1 tablespoon olive oil

Method

- Toast bread slices.
- Brush toasted bread with olive oil.
- Gently rub surface of bread with garlic clove.
- Cut each slice of toast into fingers.

If your child has to avoid dairy products, it may be tricky to provide sufficient protein. This recipe is a rich source of protein as well as some antioxidants. It is also very light on the stomach, which is important for children recovering from gastroenteritis.

Ingredients

Makes approximately:
4 serves for 1–3 year olds
3 serves for 4–7 year olds
2 serves for 8–11 year olds

250 g chicken pieces, e.g. skinless drumsticks

50 g carrots

50 g baby peas

1 small onion

1 small stalk celery with strings removed

5 g gelatine

½ teaspoon vinegar

lemon juice to drizzle

Method

- Wash the chicken pieces, and blanch in simmering salted water.
- Cook slowly for 1½–2 hours in water which just covers the pieces, adding vegetables 30 minutes before the end of cooking time.
- Remove the chicken and estimate the amount of liquid left.
- Reduce the liquid to 250 ml if necessary.
- Remove skin from the chicken, if necessary, and chop the meat finely.
- Sieve the liquid and mix with gelatine and vinegar; put aside to cool.
- Meanwhile, chop vegetables and arrange these together with the chicken meat in glass bowls or individual moulds.
- Pour the cooled stock with gelatine carefully over the chicken and the vegetables.
- Cover and allow to cool in a refrigerator.
- Serve when set, drizzled with lemon juice.

Children will love the light texture and delicious taste of these cheese balls. They are full of protein, vitamin A and zinc, and are wonderfully soft on sore throats. They contain some lactose so may not be suitable for children with gastroenteritis.

Ingredients

500 g ricotta cheese

100 g semolina

3 large eggs, separated

20 g olive margarine, monounsaturated

30 g flour, plain

Method

- Blend ricotta cheese with semolina and leave to rest for 30 minutes.
- Whip margarine with egg yolks and add salt.
- Add ricotta and semolina mixture and blend until smooth.
- Whip egg whites and fold into the mixture.
- Form mixture into small balls and roll in flour.
- Cook a few at a time, in boiling water.
- When cooked the balls should rise to the top.
- Take them out carefully and serve lightly tossed in margarine.

9
Boosting immunity with supplements

As our lifestyles become busier and time for looking after our health and that of our children becomes harder to find, we may at some time turn to supplements for help. A potential problem with this is that we may choose the wrong supplements or pay needlessly for supplements that provide no benefits. We may choose single-nutrient supplements without knowing that they can affect the amounts of other nutrients that children can absorb from their diet.

Before you reach for a supplement, bear in mind that it may do more harm than good. Dietary supplements will offer no benefit to a child whose diet is plentiful in nutrients and body stores of nutrients are normal.

Let's now consider the supplements formulated for children, especially those marketed to boost their immunity. These include vitamin and mineral supplements as well as some plant-derived supplements.

Mineral and vitamin supplements

We'll start with mineral and vitamin preparations. These usually contain a mixture of vitamins and minerals in fractions of, or in amounts several times, the recommended dietary intakes for children. The recommended dietary intakes (RDI) are set by the National Health and Medical Research Council and are the levels of essential nutrients considered adequate to meet the nutritional needs of most healthy individuals (NHMRC 1991). They are set for individual groups according to age and gender.

Mineral and vitamin supplements are a stand-by source of nutrients, mainly in synthetic form. They may come in handy when your child's diet is compromised by:

- poor eating associated with illness;
- fussy eating;
- unusual circumstances, e.g. travel, where the food is unfamiliar and your child takes a while to get used to new food choices.

When looking at mineral and vitamin supplements for their ability to boost the immune system, we must firstly consider the types and amounts of nutrients important to healthy immunity in their formulation. I checked the mineral and vitamin supplements for children and noticed differences between the brands in the quantity and quality they offer, for example, whether they are naturally derived or synthetic. So how do we know which if any of these supplements would be useful?

Let's start by looking at what we want the supplement to contain. Ideally a supplement would contain the nutrients essential for a robust immunity, but only the ones your child is deficient in (remember that research has not proven supplementation to be beneficial in children with normal body levels of nutrients).

Before you decide to have your child's blood levels tested for each nutrient you may prefer to check your child's diet, a less invasive procedure that will give a good indication of whether a deficiency is present. Keep a record of what your child eats for seven days and note any good food sources of each of the vitamin and minerals important for a strong immunity. To help assess your child's diet, refer to the best food sources for each of the nutrients important to immunity listed in Chapters 2–7. Estimate your child's average daily intake for each nutrient by adding the estimates for each out of the seven days and then dividing it by seven. If your child's average is much lower than the RDI for that nutrient then your child's body stores of this nutrient may be low. If you would like help assessing your child's diet, visit the Internet site www.nutrition4health.com.au. A portion of this website is committed to nutrient analysis and will allow you to enter the food and drinks your child consumed with a click of a button providing you with a fast and accurate nutritional analysis on a daily basis. You may also contact me via the website should you require help with your child's diet.

While you are able to get a good indication of whether or not your child is deficient in any of the nutrients by doing the above exercise, I am presently limited to providing a general guide to choosing a supplement for your child based on the following:

- food intake surveys carried out in Australian and US children;
- supplementation studies carried out in United States and developing countries.

Let's now look at the nutrients important to a healthy immunity—vitamins A, C and E; the trace minerals iron, zinc, selenium and copper; and beta carotene and flavonoids—and whether any of these are useful as supplements.

Vitamin A

Results from nutrition surveys and nutrient intake studies indicate that in a typical Western diet, children are consuming adequate amounts of vitamin A. Children on very low fat diets, however, are at a greater risk of vitamin A deficiency and supplementation may be necessary to correct low body stores of vitamin A. Unless otherwise advised by a medical practitioner, the best way to correct vitamin A deficiency is by increasing food sources rich in vitamin A (see p. 46 for excellent food sources of vitamin A). This should be accompanied by an increase in monounsaturated fat for children on very low fat diets.

Vitamin A is a fat soluble vitamin not readily regulated by the body, so if taken long term as a supplement it may build up to toxic levels. In addition, ill effects have been recorded in children given vitamin A supplement in doses of 3600 mcg retinol equivalents daily. The supplemental dose for children should always fall well below this amount and is best set by your family physician.

Vitamin C

Vitamin C is plentiful in children's diets due to relatively high consumption of fruit juices and syrups fortified with vitamin C. While reconstituted juices and syrups are not ideal sources of vitamin C—fresh fruit and vegetables being preferable—these drinks make vitamin C supplementation unnecessary in general.

In addition, it is very easy to provide children with sufficient amounts of vitamin C through diet alone. On average an orange, for example, contains 1.7 times the RDI of vitamin C for children. I consider vitamin C supplements as an unnecessary expense.

Vitamin E

Vitamin E levels have been shown to be low in the diets of children in the United States, with consistent findings across two national surveys and a few smaller studies. In Australia, reliable information is lacking with the Australian National Nutrition Survey (1995) failing to assess vitamin E intakes in children. But in light of other findings that viral infections such as the influenza virus were found to reduce tissue stores of vitamin E and the United States evidence of marginal vitamin E intakes, I think vitamin E supplementation is warranted for children who suffer from frequent infections. This is particularly true if children are consuming high levels of polyunsaturated fats (safflower and corn oils and polyunsaturated margarines) as their presence in the diet increases the need for vitamin E.

Despite some preliminary results showing that supplementation with large amounts of vitamin E is beneficial to boosting immunity, I recommend caution as there are presently no studies to document the safety of these practices in children. Instead, I recommend small supplements of vitamin E, approximating the RDI for each age group, designed to correct dietary deficiencies in children who consume marginal amounts of this vitamin.

Zinc

Studies looking at the benefits of zinc supplementation have shown mixed results, however a very well designed, community-based study in India found that zinc supplementation is beneficial in children whose zinc levels are low. Most studies that document a significant improvement in the immune response as a result of zinc supplementation use a dose of 10 mg of elemental zinc daily. This represents 222%, 167%, and 111% of the RDI for children aged 1–3, 4–7, and 8–11 years respectively. It is significant to note that most studies focused on supplementing children whose diets were extremely low in zinc. Australian children consuming a mixed diet, including lean meats, poultry and fish as well as dairy products, would have a significantly higher zinc intake and therefore a dose as high as 10 mg is unnecessary.

However, this dose may be advantageous for children on a strict vegan diet or one low in animal products as these diets are high in substances that inhibit zinc absorption, such as phytates. If your child is eating a vegan diet and regularly falls victim to infection, consider supplementing zinc at a dose of 10 mg daily for a short time as well as increasing zinc in the diet. I recommend testing your child's zinc levels before starting regular zinc supplementation at this level—remember, zinc supplementations will only be of value if your child's body stores are low and too much zinc can interfere with absorption of other minerals. Contact your doctor for further advice regarding this test.

For children who suffer from frequent opportunistic infections and who consume a mixed diet including meats, I recommend a smaller supplemental dose of 1–2 mg of zinc daily to correct possible marginal dietary deficiency. Two large national intake surveys and some smaller studies in the United States have shown that some children are not consuming the recommended amounts for zinc and the National Nutrition Survey in Australia (1995) showed similar results.

Iron

It is well established that iron and zinc compete for absorption into the body. Since both are needed for a robust immunity, a supplement minimising competition for entry into the body between these two nutrients is an added advantage and this can be achieved if the ratio of zinc to iron is kept at 2:5. So having established a helpful dose for zinc of 1–2 mg for children with a mixed diet, the corresponding dose of iron to minimise nutrient competition is 2.5–5 mg daily. For children requiring a higher dose of 10 mg of zinc to strengthen their immunity the dosage is 25 mg daily. Remember these higher doses are recommended only for children with very poor zinc and iron intakes and always after confirmation of low body levels of zinc and iron with a blood test. Even at lower levels of supplementation it is important to establish a deficiency of iron in the child's diet and body stores before commencing supplementation. Excessive iron has been shown to exacerbate infection as excess free iron in the blood is food for bacteria. I recommend caution with iron supplements for that reason.

Iron needs are greatest from 6–24 months of age and at this age it is also more difficult to obtain sufficient zinc from the diet, so supplementation with zinc and iron in small amounts may be helpful for young children who suffer frequent opportunistic infections. It is extremely important, however, to also establish eating patterns that maximise zinc and iron intakes.

Copper

The absorption of copper can be limited by zinc and iron, however if zinc and iron are given in the amounts discussed above, and providing the weight ratio of zinc to iron is kept at 2:5 respectively, copper absorption from food will not be significantly reduced. It is difficult to comment on the desirable supplemental dose of copper if any as there is no set RDI for copper in Australia, and indeed knowledge on consumption levels in children is lacking.

Selenium

As the selenium content of crops is largely dependant on the selenium content of the soil where they are grown, selenium consumption will differ widely and routine selenium supplementation is not desirable.

It is also difficult to establish whether or not children are consuming sufficient amounts of selenium. Studies looking at children's intakes of selenium must take into account the variable selenium content of the plant food sources in children's diets and as these may have been grown in widely different geographical locations with significant differences in the selenium content of the soil, using standard tables for selenium content of foods is inadequate. The selenium content in Australian soils generally is not considered low by world standards and selenium deficiency due to poor soil content is not considered to be a public health issue. For these reasons I do not recommend selenium supplementation in children to boost immunity.

If you are growing your own vegetables and would like to test the selenium content of your soil, you can do so by submitting a 500 g sample to Sydney Environmental and Soil Laboratory. You can contact them via email at sesl@sesl.com.au.

Beta carotene and flavonoids

Beta carotene can be easily obtained from the diet via green, orange and yellow fruit and vegetables. These are usually well liked by children and supplementation of beta carotene is unnecessary. I am not aware of research which supports supplementation with beta carotene in children.

Similarly, flavonoids are present in a variety of fruit, vegetables and other plant foods. Including supplements with specific flavonoids can give us a false sense of security and undermine our efforts to include more fruit and vegetables in our children's diets, which offer by far a better variety of flavonoids. In addition, the processing of supplements, such as the drying of plant extracts containing flavonoids, is bound to destroy some of the beneficial antioxidant properties of flavonoids.

In summary, supplementation with vitamin E, zinc and iron may be beneficial for some children suffering frequent opportunistic infections, and particularly for children with vegetarian or vegan diets, high in polyunsaturated fats and low in meat and dairy products. From 6–24 months of age is a crucial stage in childhood development when iron and zinc needs are not easily met by the diet. Checking your child's diet to ensure it supplies adequate amounts of these nutrients is essential at this time. If you suspect your child is not consuming adequate amounts of iron or zinc, consult a qualified dietitian nutritionist or your family physician for further advice.

Echinacea

Echinacea has become popular as a natural cure for colds and other upper respiratory infections. Echinacea species, or purple coneflower, has long been used for its medicinal properties including relief of symptoms associated with the common cold. It was first used by Native Americans, followed by the European settlers who cultivated the plant after taking it back to Europe. Unknowingly, the Europeans took back a different species called *Echinacea purpurea,* which turned out to be just as useful. Today, both species, *Echinacea purpurea* and *Echinacea angustifolia,* as well as a third called *Echinacea pallida* are commonly referred to as echinacea. Echinacea supplements may contain all three species, a combination of them, or just one of the species.

Echinacea extracts are believed to have an immuno-stimulating effect, which makes them useful for other upper respiratory conditions as well as the common cold. A number of studies have reported enhanced phagocytosis, that is, a speeding up of the immune cells that gobble up foreign matter, including bacteria. In addition, antibacterial and antiviral properties have been noted in echinacea extracts. Various compounds, rather than a single substance, are thought responsible for the beneficial actions on the immune system, including polysaccharides and flavonoids.

There are significant differences in the chemical composition and, therefore, the medicinal properties of the three species of echinacea, and even between the parts of each plant. And the way in which the bio-active molecules are extracted makes a difference to their potency. It seems that alcohol extraction of the molecules that stimulate the immune system destroys their beneficial properties, while water extraction does not. To date, studies looking at the effects of echinacea on the immune system, although numerous, have failed to find a uniform measure of the active ingredients in the plant. This makes comparison between studies very difficult.

A recent report in the *Journal of Family Practice* (1999), however, collated the results of all published studies, books and book chapters on the medicinal use of echinacea and concluded that 'echinacea may be beneficial for the early treatment of acute upper respiratory infections' but 'there is very little evidence supporting the prolonged use of echinacea for the prevention of upper respiratory infections'. From the scientific trials carried out on echinacea it appears that it is safe and can be effective in reducing the severity and duration of the common cold but is not effective in preventing the onsets of colds and flu.

Although echinacea is considered a well tolerated medicinal

herb, as with all other medicinal plants the possibility of an allergic reaction can't be ruled out. In cases where a child suffers from allergic conditions like asthma and rhinitis, the chances of an allergic reaction to echinacea increase. The risks in children haven't been documented but a study in adults showed that 19% of adults with asthma and allergic rhinitis also reacted to echinacea extract. It is best to see your doctor to exclude the possibility of allergy if you are thinking of starting your child on echinacea supplements.

For maximum benefit, echinacea supplements should be taken early in the course of a cold or flu, taken several times a day, and discontinued as symptoms clear. As the content of leaves, stems and roots varies greatly in their chemical composition, and the beneficial effect on the immune system is most probably due to more than one compound, whole-plant extracts would appear more useful than isolated ingredients. Finally, long-term safety of the plant is not documented, and no studies have looked into the safety of using echinacea in the treatment of upper respiratory infections in children.

Garlic

Garlic is a popular supplement used by many to prevent or treat upper respiratory infections. The ancient Egyptians, Greeks, Romans, Indians and Chinese have cultivated garlic for its medicinal properties, including for the treatment of wounds and infections. In 1858 Louis Pasteur showed that garlic has antibacterial properties, and more recent research supports his discovery. Garlic juices have been shown to kill many fungi and numerous strains of bacteria.

The active ingredient responsible for these beneficial effects is *allicin*. Allicin forms when the garlic cloves are crushed and a natural substance called alliin is combined with an enzyme, allinase, which converts alliin to allicin. The crushing of the garlic releases the enzyme allinase from tiny vesicles inside the garlic clove, preventing the conversion of alliin to allicin in intact garlic cloves. Allicin is easily identified by the strong odour of garlic. Fresh garlic preparations contain the highest amounts of the active ingredient allicin and other beneficial compounds including antioxidants.

There are many garlic supplements, all claiming to have health benefits without the unpleasant odour. Supplements containing the active antibacterial ingredients can be very useful for children who dislike the strong smell and taste of garlic, and particularly for young children who may have problems digesting fresh garlic. While cooking reduces the strong odour and makes garlic easier to digest, it also destroys allinase, the enzyme responsible for producing allicin. In effect, cooking destroys most of the antibacterial effects of garlic.

Most studies report a positive effect of garlic preparations as long as they deliver a sufficient dose of allicin, or alliin that can be converted to allicin in the body. For this the enzyme allinase is necessary. The enzyme is inactivated, however, by heat, oxygen and water and this accounts for the fact that cooked garlic (as well as some garlic preparations) does not have such a strong odour as raw garlic, nor are its medicinal effects nearly as powerful.

Steam distillation and other high-temperature water extractions are thought to contain almost none of the beneficial compounds. Gelatine capsules containing oil, are usually the end product of distillation.

Dried garlic does contain the active compound alliin and small amounts of allicin. The enzyme allinase may be present in dried garlic that has been dried at low temperatures, but this enzyme is unstable in the presence of acid. When dried garlic is consumed and reaches the stomach, the allinase is destroyed by stomach acid, so not much alliin is converted to allicin. To overcome this difficulty some companies have produced dry garlic powder caplets enclosed in a protective coat, which allows the garlic supplement to travel to the intestine before being absorbed. This prevents the destruction of allinase in the stomach and allows for the conversion of alliin to allicin.

Garlic supplements designed for children include dry bulb preparations in chewable, fruit-flavoured tablets, claiming to be odourless, and freeze-dried powder in a tablet form to be swallowed. In addition, garlic oil extracted from fresh garlic and packaged in a gelatin capsule, which is not odourless, is also available. This type of preparation is marketed as suitable for children over six years of age.

Despite the appeal of processed garlic preparations, fresh garlic is a less expensive and more effective antimicrobial agent. Used in moderation, the smell and taste of garlic is not overpowering, even for young children.

Probiotics

Finally, let's look at probiotics. Supplemental doses of probiotics may be beneficial for a few weeks following a course of antibiotics in children to help replenish friendly bacteria in the digestive tract. They are particularly helpful following infectious diarrhoea and the development of transient lactose intolerance when milk-based probiotics are not suitable as they contain lactose. They should not be taken long-term. The probiotic supplements available for children include tablets of *Lactobacillus acidophilus* as well as combinations of *Lactobacillus acidophilus* and *Bifidobacterium lactis*. Both *Lactobacillus acidophilus* and *Bifidobacterium lactis* are helpful to reestablish a healthy microflora. When purchasing probiotic supplements, always check age recommendations.

To be of benefit, the daily dosage of probiotics must contain at least 10^9 of viable organisms daily, with 10^{10} being preferable. Note that some yoghurts contain 10^{10} of viable *Lactobacillus rhemnosus* GG—shown to be effective in shortening the duration of antibiotic-related diarrhoea—in a 150 ml serving. As yoghurt is low in lactose, it may be well tolerated by children with acute diarrhoea accompanied by reduced tolerance of foods containing lactose.

10
Exercise for good immunity

A moderate amount of regular exercise strengthens the immune system, and has been shown to reduce the incidence of upper respiratory infections. Moderate aerobic exercise—40 minutes five times a week—showed a significant effect on reducing the frequency of the common cold. These beneficial effects on the immune system are thought to be due to a faster, better performance by the natural killer cells—the fighter cells involved in the first-line defence against bacteria and viruses. Naturally, a faster response by these fighter cells, resulting in faster destruction of the invading viruses, is a better guarantee against viral infection.

Several studies comparing the number of natural killer cells before and after exercise programs show that the numbers go up significantly after moderate physical activity as compared to sedentary individuals or individuals who undertake strenuous regular exercise. A study of a small group of children in Russia showed that moderate training, in this case regular swimming, improved children's resistance to infections.

Are Australian children fit?

What is the right amount of exercise for children? Are Australian children sufficiently active? There is no accepted answer to the first question nor any formal guidelines for children available for parents to follow. There is not enough information available for us to know how fit is fit enough for children. The minimum recommendation for schoolage children, reported by the United States Public Health Service in *American Family Physician* (November 1994) is 20–30 minutes of vigorous exercise at least three times weekly.

Another way to assess whether your children are sufficiently active is to appraise their weight. If your child is overweight or obese, it is likely that they are not getting enough exercise. It is estimated that, in Australia, 25% of children are overweight or obese. This correlates quite well with an estimate of 20% of children who are inactive, based on the NSW Schools Fitness and Physical Activity Survey carried out in 1997. Based on these figures we can say that approximately one in four Australian children are overweight and are unlikely to be taking sufficient exercise. The immune system of these children misses out on the benefits of regular exercise and is also placed at risk by the deleterious effects of excess weight, particularly obesity brought on by poor eating habits.

In the absence of established activity guidelines for parents in Australia, some recommendations for physical activity for children were published in the *Medical Journal of Australia* in August 2000:

- Provide daily opportunities for children to be active, in a variety of ways, in a safe environment.
- Avoid driving children on short trips when walking is possible.
- Limit the time children are allowed to spend in sedentary recreation such as watching television and playing computer games—say, 30 minutes a day.

- Support children's development of the fundamental movement skills by playing games with them, encouraging them to play sport, and asking your child's school to implement the Fundamental Movement Skills curriculum.

You can obtain more information regarding the Fundamental Movement Skills curriculum by visiting its website at: www.curriculumsupport.nsw.edu.au.

Putting guidelines into practice

- Consider community clubs, teams and associations; encourage friends to visit and play; take children to a park, pool or beach; find somewhere safe for them to ride a bike.
- Walk your child to school or see if it is possible to organise 'walking buses' where a small group of children is supervised by an adult.
- Set an example by being active yourself and involving your children.
- Start with fundamental motor skills like throwing and catching a ball.
- Encourage your child to take part in a variety of activities.
- For children who are more serious about a sport, avoid early 'specialisation' in one sport as it can lead to overuse injuries.

To prevent child injuries related to physical activity

- Make sure your child does warm-up and cooling-down exercises.
- Ensure your child is active in a safe environment.
- Provide adequate sports equipment, particularly protective equipment if needed.
- Supply comfortable shoes to prevent blistering of feet.
- Provide adequate fluid to prevent dehydration and heatstroke (Sports Medicine Australia recommends that active children drink a glass of fluid 45 minutes before exercise and continue to drink an additional 75–100 ml of fluid every 20 minutes during exercise).
- Provide a drink after exercise. Choose water or sports drinks if particularly thirsty and active, as they are more quickly absorbed.
- Prevent sunburn if playing out in the sun—avoid physical activity in the middle of the day during summer.
- Emphasise fair play and fun.

Source: Adapted from 'Recommendations for nutrition and physical activity for Australian children', *Medical Journal of Australia* 7 August 2000, v. 173, supplement.

Encouraging children to be active

Young children don't need motivation to be active. It is part of their nature to move about endlessly, involving their young bodies in sporadic running, jumping, spinning, rolling and twisting. They seem to have endless energy and to gain real enjoyment from physical activity. There is usually no need to increase the activity levels of children up to the age of three. All that's necessary is a safe and happy environment in which to be physically active.

This happy involvement in physical activity wanes as children get older, and nowhere more quickly than in today's Western society where social and personal factors often bring physical activity in older children to a halt. The main reasons for this trend include the physical passivity of watching television, sedentary involvement in computer games, and in many cases lack of time for family physical activities because both parents are working full time to support a young family.

To counteract these negative influences, many older children must be actively motivated to exercise. Some clear goals and a game plan are handy. Don't set your expectations too high—if your child has been sedentary or, particularly, is overweight, start gently. Your goal is to introduce exercise into your child's life. Create a pleasant and enjoyable experience, as this in itself will motivate your child to have another go. When you have established your child's interest in a given activity, work on nurturing that interest and develop it into a routine.

Remember that, in children there is no place for the 'no gain without pain' attitude to sport. A 30-minute aerobic workout is quite inappropriate in children starting to exercise—they would refuse any further offers after half an hour of panting, sweating and moaning. It would turn into a bad memory, and eventually fuel a return to the television screen with a packet of chips and a reluctance to do anything physical in the future. Starting with an easy, fun activity is essential, especially for a child who is overweight.

Try to involve the child in activities enjoyed by other members of the family, but take care to avoid competition or teasing among siblings or peers. Applaud any improvement and initiate the physical activities over and over again until they become part of the child's routine. An activity that children enjoy will stay with them well into adulthood. Studies have shown that exercise habits established during childhood predict exercise habits in adulthood.

When you first set out to involve your children in physical activity, remember to evaluate their progress. If things don't go as planned the first few times, and your child is still reluctant to take part in exercise, keep in mind these points outlined by Thomas Rowland (*Exercise and Children's Health,* Human Kinetics Books, Champaign, Ill., 1990). The motivating forces for a child to take part in exercise are:

- fun;
- success, i.e. they should feel they are doing well;
- peer support;
- family participation;
- variety;
- enthusiastic leader;
- freedom.

The turnoffs are:

- discomfort;
- failure;
- embarrassment;
- competition;
- boredom;
- injuries;
- regimentation.

Fun physical activities for children

What is fun and games for one child may not be for another so it is important to know what your child likes or may like when initiating physical activity. Even very sedentary children usually have something in mind that they wouldn't mind doing or at least are willing to try. If you don't get a response from your child, suggest something yourself—maybe walking through a zoo or park to start with.

Walking

Walking is particularly suited to young children or to older children with little previous physical activity. Because it is less intense than other forms of exercise, walking allows for socialising as well. You can 'catch up' with your children on a walk, you may find they will enjoy telling you things and you may cover some ground both physically and emotionally. Walking outdoors allows children, as well as you, to catch up with the environment and this is refreshing. Competition, insufficient skills and a fear of failing at social sports are avoided. Walking gives every child a sense of achievement. And walks can be made even more enjoyable by planning trips to the zoo or museums, and using the walking tracks in local national parks.

Things to remember when venturing out on a walk are comfortable shoes, and cotton clothes to reduce sweating. For heavy children put some talcum powder between their thighs and under their arms to prevent a rash, especially in warm weather.

Swimming

Being in the water is fun for children who know how to swim. It is also fun to dive and it feels very good to cool off in the water in summer. Even youngsters who haven't yet mastered the strokes that will allow them to swim will enjoy playing in the waves supervised by an adult or older sibling. Encouraging your kids to frolic about in the waves or in the local pool gets them familiar with water and they begin to enjoy being in it. You can enrol your child in community swimming lessons to learn how to swim or to improve their strokes and stamina.

Swimming is good for all children and particularly benefits children who are overweight for it has none of the stresses experienced in weight-bearing exercises. Watch out for ear infections, which can be prevented if your child wears earplugs (and of course by looking after your child's immune system).

Cycling

Riding a bike seems to be the favourite of all sports. Even sedentary TV-loving youngsters claim to have jumped on a bike. Children like to cycle because, unlike walking, it gets them from A to B fast and the speed gives them a thrill. It is relatively easy providing you don't choose to go uphill.

There are some great cycling tracks available for weekend enjoyment by the entire family. Things to remember are helmets and road safety rules. Some children, boys in particular, get a kick out of fixing their bikes as well as riding them.

Activities for overweight children

For very inactive children, complicated by obesity, it is important to start very gently. You could involve your child in more household chores with you, remembering to make them fun, of course. Play outside with your child at throwing and catching activities, making a point of the child fetching the ball if they drop it! Buying a dog can be the best incentive for the much needed exercise in this group of children. Walking with a small puppy is so much more fun than doing the paces as a chore. And just throwing a ball for the dog and running around after it in the garden for an hour or so a day does a lot of good.

Buying a dog is a big responsibility but, with older children who are excited at the idea, it is easy to foster duty-sharing. You want them to become more physically active and this is a golden opportunity to initiate walking the dog in the neighbourhood and other active fun and games. Remember that puppies, like very young children, love to move around and their enjoyment spreads to children who are then so much more likely to join in.

Involving your child in social or competitive sports

There are lots of social sports with more structured training regimes. When thinking about enrolling in these sports consider your child's previous activity level and their fitness, general health and attitude to sport. Discuss these details with your child and consider a visit to your doctor for further discussions if you and your child are considering a strenuous sport or one that involves contact and collisions.

Tables 10.1 and 10.2 may help when deciding on the type of sport to enrol your child in.

Table 10.1

Classification of sports according to contact level

Contact/collision	**Limited contact/impact**
Boxing	Baseball
Field hockey	Basketball
Football	Cycling
Ice hockey	Handball
Martial arts	Roller skating
Soccer	Softball
Wrestling	Squash
	Volleyball

Source: American Academy of Paediatrics, Committee of Sports Medicine and Fitness. 'Recommendations for participation in sports', *Paediatrics* 1988; 81:737–39.

Table 10.2

Classification of sports according to level of activity

Strenuous	**Moderately strenuous**	**Non-strenuous**
Aerobic dancing	Badminton	Archery
Fencing	Table tennis	Golf
Running		
Swimming		
Tennis		
Track		

Source: American Academy of Paediatrics, Committee of Sports Medicine and Fitness. 'Recommendations for participation in sports', *Paediatrics* 1988; 81:737–39.

11

Balancing children's menus to boost immunity

Having looked at your child's requirements for the immunity-boosting nutrients, and the whereabouts of these nutrients in the diet, we now look at how to go about planning a nutritionally balanced menu—a menu that includes adequate amounts of these nutrients as well as meeting the recommendations for all other nutrients in your child's diet.

Carry out a quick review of the minimum food serves from the five food groups, as recommended for children in the three different age groups, by looking back at Table 1.1 (p. 12). The guidelines in Table 1.1 give us a reasonable idea of the amounts and types of foods your child needs to consume from each of the five food groups. We now need to turn these guidelines into more specific food choices, taking into account the specific developmental stage of your child, depending on age.

Food choices for children aged 1–3 years

By now your child should be drinking from a cup. He or she has some teeth and will develop a full set of twenty teeth so chewing will be possible and varied textures from very soft to crisp are appropriate. Children are also able to feed themselves, with a degree of charming clumsiness to start with, progressing to the more skilled older toddler. Older toddlers are able to enjoy most family meals and eat a wide variety of foods, although spicy and fried food should be avoided.

Milk remains important and your child should continue to drink about 600 ml of whole milk daily. Cheese or yoghurt can be substituted for milk. Meat should be tender and easily chewed for toddlers: lean meat loaf, well done pot roasts, casseroles, soft chicken pieces and fish. When cooking fish take care to remove all bones. Eggs and cheese are often toddlers' favourite items as they are easy to chew and swallow. For children, don't limit eggs to two a week—this recommendation may be suitable for some adults, not growing children who need extra protein and nutrients for healthy development. Introducing a wide variety of fruit and vegetables, breads and cereals as well as water to your child is important at this stage for they help to establish healthy eating habits for a lifetime.

During the toddler years growth slows down in comparison to infancy, so expect appetites to decrease a little. Providing six meals a day is important: three main meals and three nourishing snacks help to maintain good nutrition.

Some foods are not suitable for toddlers and young children because they are difficult to chew and swallow and may cause your child to choke. The following are not suitable until the age of five:

- raw carrots;
- raw celery;
- corn kernels;
- chips;
- hard-to-chew meats;

- nuts, unless ground;
- peanut butter from a spoon (sticky and difficult to swallow);
- popcorn;
- small hard lollies;
- dried sultanas or raisins;
- other small, round foods.

Food choices for children aged 4–7 years

In this age group children start to show curiosity about foods and are often happy to take part in preparing meals. This is a good time to involve your children in preparing nutritious foods to nurture good eating habits. By this stage your child is well and truly enjoying foods with the rest of the family. I do recommend caution, however, with the following items: heavily spiced meals, fatty meats or cold cuts, pickles based on vinegar as they are very high in salt and, finally, bought paté or fresh soft cheeses, because of the possibility of contamination with listeria.

Five to six meals daily remain important for children in this age group. Milk should be offered whole, not fat-reduced until the age of five, and can be continued for longer if your child is not overweight. Advice for offering a wide variety of foods to toddlers remains valid in this age group, particularly fresh fruit and vegetables.

Food choices for children aged 8–11 years

For older children the number of meals can be reduced to four, sometimes five, daily. Breakfast is a must in order to obtain sufficient nutrients daily. Research shows that skipping breakfast brings about poorer cognitive performance, resulting in poorer grades at school. Eating morning tea at recess during the school week is important and ideally should constitute a nutritious snack. Afternoon tea at home offers a chance to bring the balance back to a more nutritious one if school lunch or break snack lacked variety (due to less nutritious canteen choices or peer pressure to eat processed foods). Fruit, breads and dairy foods make good snacks for the afternoon.

It is important to encourage your child to eat meals that include lean meats, poultry and fish as part of a healthy and varied diet. These sources of protein can be varied from time to time by giving eggs, cheese, nuts or legumes. Milk and dairy products may now be fat-reduced. Eating a wide variety of fruits and vegetables as well as a range of grains and cereals is important to meet energy needs as well as immunity-boosting nutrients.

Sample menus rich in immunity-boosting nutrients.

After this brief look at suitable food choices and meal patterns for children in each age group, it is now time to browse through some balanced daily menus. Each daily menu meets at least the daily recommended dietary intake (RDI) for each immunity-boosting nutrient, as well as including other nutrients important to your child's health. Each daily menu includes three main meals and three nourishing snacks. For older children it may be more practical to provide four or five meals, in which case one of the snacks can be omitted and the morning snack made bigger.

For younger children, dilute fruit juice half-half with water. For all children, encourage drinking water and avoid offering soft drinks and sweetened artificially flavoured cordial.

As you look through the menus you will notice that some dishes are printed in *italics*—this means that you will find the recipe for that dish in this book (see recipe index). These recipes were chosen for their high content of immunity-boosting nutrients. Have a go at some of the recipes—you may like to make them into meals for the entire family. The amounts of ingredients will often feed a family of four. The serving size of meals will vary, depending on your child's age, activity level and build.

Breakfast
Cereal and milk
Stewed peaches

Morning Tea
Peanut butter and banana toast
Milk

Lunch
Carrot and orange soup
Ham roll-arounds

Afternoon Tea
Raspberry smoothie

Dinner
Tuna casserole

Supper
Chocolate and pear pudding

Breakfast
Cereal with milk
Baked beans on toast
Fresh pawpaw

Morning Tea
Pikelet with *fruit and nut spread*
Milk

Lunch
Vegetable curry with basmati rice

Afternoon Tea
Yoghurt
Fruit salad

Dinner
Spinach lasagne
Freshly squeezed orange juice

Supper
Hot chocolate

Breakfast
Honeyed porridge
Scrambled egg on toast
Freshly squeezed orange juice

Morning Tea
Fruit muffin
Milk

Lunch
Cauliflower cheese soup
Bread roll

Afternoon Tea
Strawberries and custard

Dinner
Veal meatballs
Mashed potato
Carrots
Green beans

Supper
Fruit smoothie

Breakfast
Scrambled egg with ham on toast
Freshly squeezed orange juice

Morning Tea
English muffin, toasted
Tuna paste
Milk

Lunch
Fried rice

Afternoon Tea
Fruit salad
Vanilla yoghurt

Dinner
Pork and apple meat loaf
Broccoli
Carrot
Mashed potato

Supper
Tender prunes and custard

Breakfast
Cereal with milk, sprinkled with almond meal
Strawberries

Morning Tea
Asparagus frittata
Freshly squeezed orange juice

Lunch
Chicken and sweet corn soup
Cheese and tomato on toast

Afternoon Tea
Fruit muffin
Milk

Dinner
Mango fish
Yellow squash
Broccoli
Rice

Supper
Fruit salad and ice-cream

Breakfast
Egg tomato moulds on toast
Milk

Morning Tea
Whole-wheat blueberry muffins
Milk

Lunch
Avocado, turkey and tomato sandwiches
Freshly squeezed orange juice

Afternoon Tea
Fresh fruit

Dinner
Creamy chicken pasta

Supper
Dried fruit and nut compote and custard

Breakfast
Sardines on toast
Freshly squeezed orange juice

Morning Tea
Honey cinnamon crumpet
Milk

Lunch
Mini baked potato with avocado stuffing

Afternoon Tea
Yoghurt
Banana

Dinner
Beef stir-fry and rice

Supper
Apricot crumble
Milk

Breakfast
Cereal and milk
Banana and strawberries

Morning Tea
Peanut butter sandwich
Milk

Lunch
Bean hotpot with vegetables and couscous
Freshly squeezed orange juice

Afternoon Tea
Baked ricotta molehills

Dinner
Chicken with apricots

Supper
Hot chocolate

Breakfast
Cheese on toast
Milk
Apple pieces

Morning Tea
Scone and jam
Milk

Lunch
Sweet corn omelette
Freshly squeezed orange juice

Afternoon Tea
Avocado, ham and tomato sandwiches

Dinner
Mexican beef burritos

Supper
Melon plate

Breakfast
Baked beans on a crumpet
Milk
Cut-up kiwi fruit and strawberries

Morning Tea
Whole-wheat blueberry muffin
Milk

Lunch
Mediterranean chickpeas
Freshly squeezed orange juice

Afternoon Tea
Banana smoothie (see *raspberry smoothie*)

Dinner
Fishcakes
Mashed potato
Carrots and zucchini

Supper
Creamed rice

Breakfast
Green and gold eggs
Toast soldiers
Milk
Fresh pear

Morning Tea
Fruit muffin
Milk

Lunch
Minestrone soup
Cheese on toast
Freshly squeezed orange juice

Afternoon Tea
Fruit salad

Dinner
Beefburger deluxe

Supper
Apple strudel
Vanilla ice-cream with pecan nuts

Breakfast
Cereal and milk
Cut-up banana

Morning Tea
Yoghurt
Melon plate

Lunch
Macaroni and vegetable medley
Freshly squeezed orange juice

Afternoon Tea
Apple cinnamon scones
Milk

Dinner
Satay chicken on a bed of rice

Supper
Raisin or jam wholemeal toast
Milk

Breakfast
Honeyed porridge
Freshly squeezed orange juice

Morning Tea
Fruit muffin
Milk

Lunch
Ham roll-arounds

Afternoon Tea
Fruit salad and yoghurt

Dinner
Cheesy fish bake

Supper
Tender prunes and custard

Breakfast
Potato rosti
Milk
Fresh fruit salad

Morning Tea
Peanut butter on toasted crumpet
Freshly squeezed orange juice

Lunch
Tofu burgers
Broccoli
Carrots
Mashed potato

Afternoon Tea
Vanilla yoghurt and plain biscuit

Dinner
Lamb chops
Vegetable mix, steamed
Mashed potato

Supper
Hot chocolate

Glossary

antibody A protein produced in the body in response to invasion by a foreign agent.

antioxidant A substance that in small amounts prevents damage to cell components by neutralising free radicals. Antioxidants are plentiful in fruit, vegetables, legumes and some cereals.

B lymphocyte A class of cells of the adaptive immune system that become activated in the presence of foreign bodies. Once activated they produce antibodies that help to destroy specific foreign microorganisms.

beta carotene The best known of the carotenoids, beta carotene is converted into vitamin A in the body. It is present in yellow and orange coloured fruit and yellow and dark green vegetables. Beta carotene has antioxidant properties.

carotenoids A large group of compounds found in yellow and dark green vegetables and fruits. Carotenoids have antioxidant properties.

cholesterol A waxy substance essential to the function of the nervous and endocrine systems. Excessive amounts of cholesterol in the blood may lead to fatty deposits in the arteries and increase the likelihood of heart disease.

cytokine A group of related proteins that are produced by the body's cells in response to infection and which coordinate the immune system's attack against infectious agents.

epithelial cell Cells that form membranes lining the bodily cavities and canals that lead to the outside, for example the respiratory and the digestive tracts. Mucous membranes formed from epithelial cells line many tracts and structures of the body and act as a physical barrier to microorganisms.

fad A temporary increase in the demand for certain foods, sometimes to the exclusion of all other foods. Fads are a natural part of childhood.

flavonoids A specific group of plant compounds, flavonoids are best known for their being powerful plant antioxidants due to their chemical structure. Flavonoids are particularly plentiful in fruit and vegetables as well as tea.

free radical An unstable molecule capable of damaging cell components and DNA. Free radicals are formed in the body as byproducts of metabolism.

lactose A sugar found in milk, including cow and goat's milk. Some children have lactose intolerance, a condition where they cannot digest lactose, and may experience bloating, nausea and sometimes vomiting after consuming milk or other dairy products containing lactose.

legumes Plants from the single family *Leguminosae* or *Fabaceae* (peanuts, dried peas, beans and lentils). Legumes are an important source of protein in vegan and macrobiotic diets. Some, such as soybeans, are very good sources of flavonoids.

macrophage A type of white blood cell that can ingest and destroy bacteria. Alveolar macrophages form the first line of defence in the lung and are very important in the fight against respiratory infections.

mast cell A type of white blood cell involved in hypersensitivity and allergic reactions. Mast cells are scattered throughout the connective tissues of the body, particularly just beneath the surface of the skin near capillaries and lymphatic vessels.

metabolism A group of chemical reactions that take place within living cells deriving energy mainly from fats and carbohydrates. Necessary for maintaining vital processes, repairing cell components and for the manufacture of new organic materials.

microbe An invasive foreign body also referred to as micro-organism.

microgram A unit of measure (one millionth of a gram) used to specify small amounts of certain nutrients, for example, selenium.

natural killer cell A specialised white blood cell that has the ability to recognise and destroy virus-infected and tumour cells.

neutrophil The most abundant type of white blood cell. Neutrophils play a major role in the recognition and killing of microorganisms.

obesity A condition where excessive body fat is present and weight is at least 20% above the ideal body weight. Obesity is usually caused by the consumption of more kilojoules than the body can use.

oxalate A compound found in plants such as legumes. Oxalates can reduce the absorption of iron and calcium by forming insoluble mineral salts.

phagocyte A white blood cell capable of ingesting microbes such as bacteria, dead tissue cells and foreign particles.

phagocytosis A process by which white blood cells called phagocytes ingest or engulf other cells or particles.

phytate A plant compound found mainly in unprocessed cereals that have the ability to bind iron and zinc, as well as other minerals, making them less available for absorption.

polypeptide A compound containing two or more amino acids. Many hormones, immunity-stimulating substances and other compounds that participate in the metabolic functions of living organisms are polypeptides.

polyphenol A major class of compounds found in plants including flavonoids. Polyphenols have strong antioxidant properties.

probiotics Friendly strains of bacteria that help to maintain a healthy intestinal flora by preventing harmful bacteria from taking a foothold. May be beneficial in stimulating the immune system in its fight against microbes.

T lymphocyte A type of lymphocyte (cell of the adaptive immune system) that becomes activated in the presence of foreign bodies. Once activated they produce immunity-stimulating molecules that coordinate the activities of the immune system to destroy invading microorganisms. These cells work closely with B lymphocytes.

tannin Plant chemical widely present in fruit, tea, chocolate, legumes and some cereals. Tannins reduce the digestibility of proteins by forming insoluble complexes that resist digestion by enzymes.

vitamin A substance essential for normal health and growth in humans. Vitamins constitute a small fraction of the diet ranging from 0.00002 per cent to 0.005 per cent.

white blood cell A cell of the immune system present in the blood, also known as a leukocyte. Its chief function is to protect the body against microorganisms causing disease.

Conversions

1 cup = 250 ml		1 teaspoon = 5 ml	
¼ cup = 60 ml		½ teaspoon = 2.5 ml	
⅓ cup = 80 ml		1 tablespoon = 20 ml	
½ cup = 125 ml			

Mass (weight)

Metric	Imperial	Metric	Imperial
15 g	½ oz	315 g	10 oz
30 g	1 oz	345 g	11 oz
60 g	2 oz	375 g	12 oz (¾ lb)
90 g	3 oz	410 g	13 oz
120 g	4 oz (¼ lb)	440 g	14 oz
155 g	5 oz	470 g	15 oz
185 g	6 oz	500 g (0.5 kg)	16 oz (1 lb)
220 g	7 oz	750 g	24 oz (1½ lb)
250 g	8 oz (½ lb)	1000 g (1 kg)	32 oz (2 lb)
280 g	9 oz		

Liquids

Metric	Cup	Imperial
30 ml		1 fl oz
60 ml	¼ cup	2 fl oz
90 ml		3 fl oz
120 ml	½ cup	4 fl oz
150 ml		5 fl oz (¼ pint)
200 ml	¾ cup	6 fl oz
250 ml	1 cup	8 fl oz
300 ml	1¼ cups	10 fl oz (½ pint)
375 ml	1½ cups	12 fl oz
425 ml	1¾ cups	14 fl oz
475 ml		15 fl oz
500 ml	2 cups	16 fl oz
600 ml	2½ cups	20 fl oz (1 pint)

Index of recipes

Index of topics